RETIRED NURSE

ADULT COLORING BOOK

Enjoying this book?

Please leave a review because we would love to know your thoughts, feedback, and opinions to create better paper products for you!

Thank you so much for your support.

Copyright © 2020. All rights reserved.

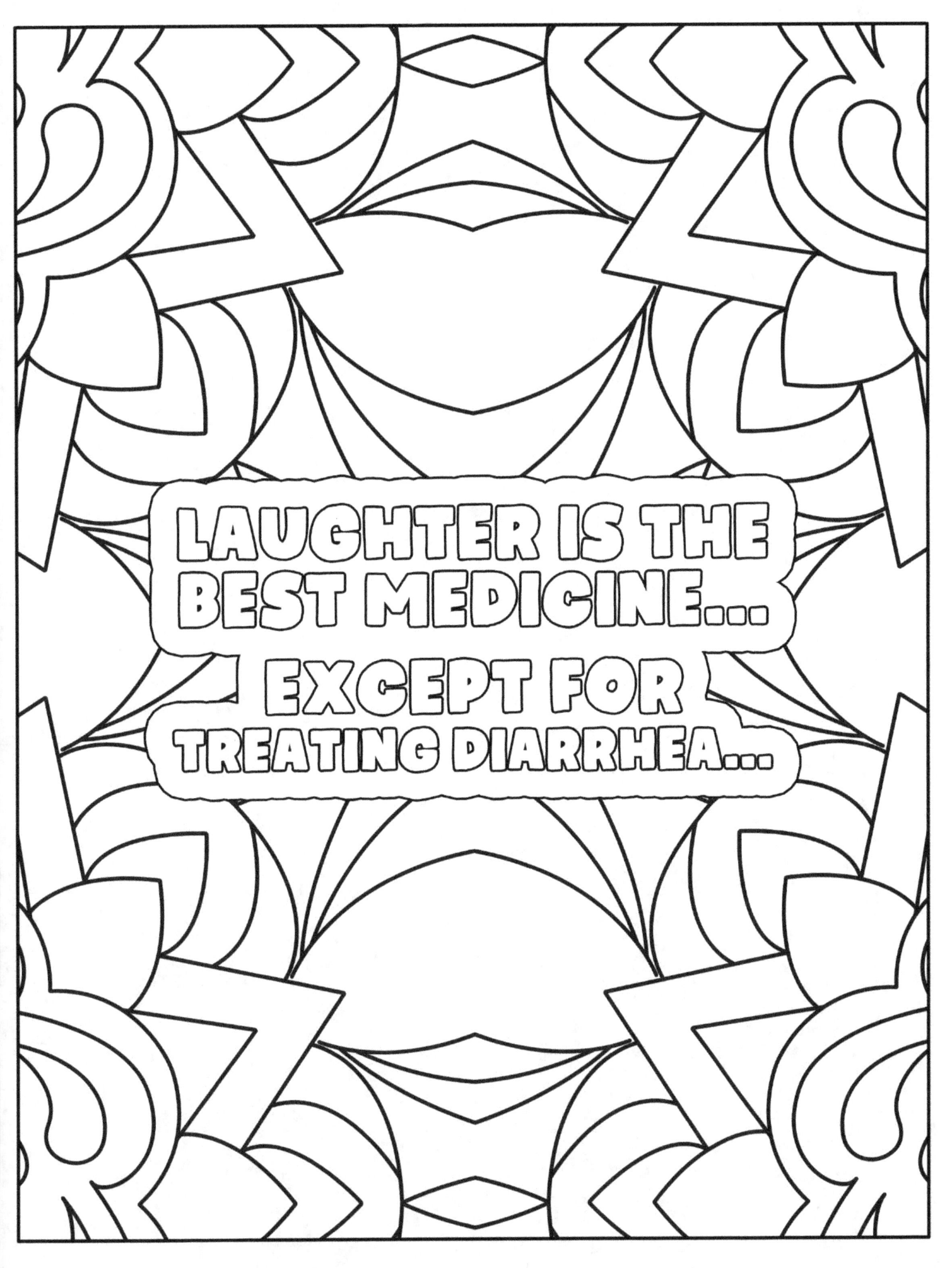

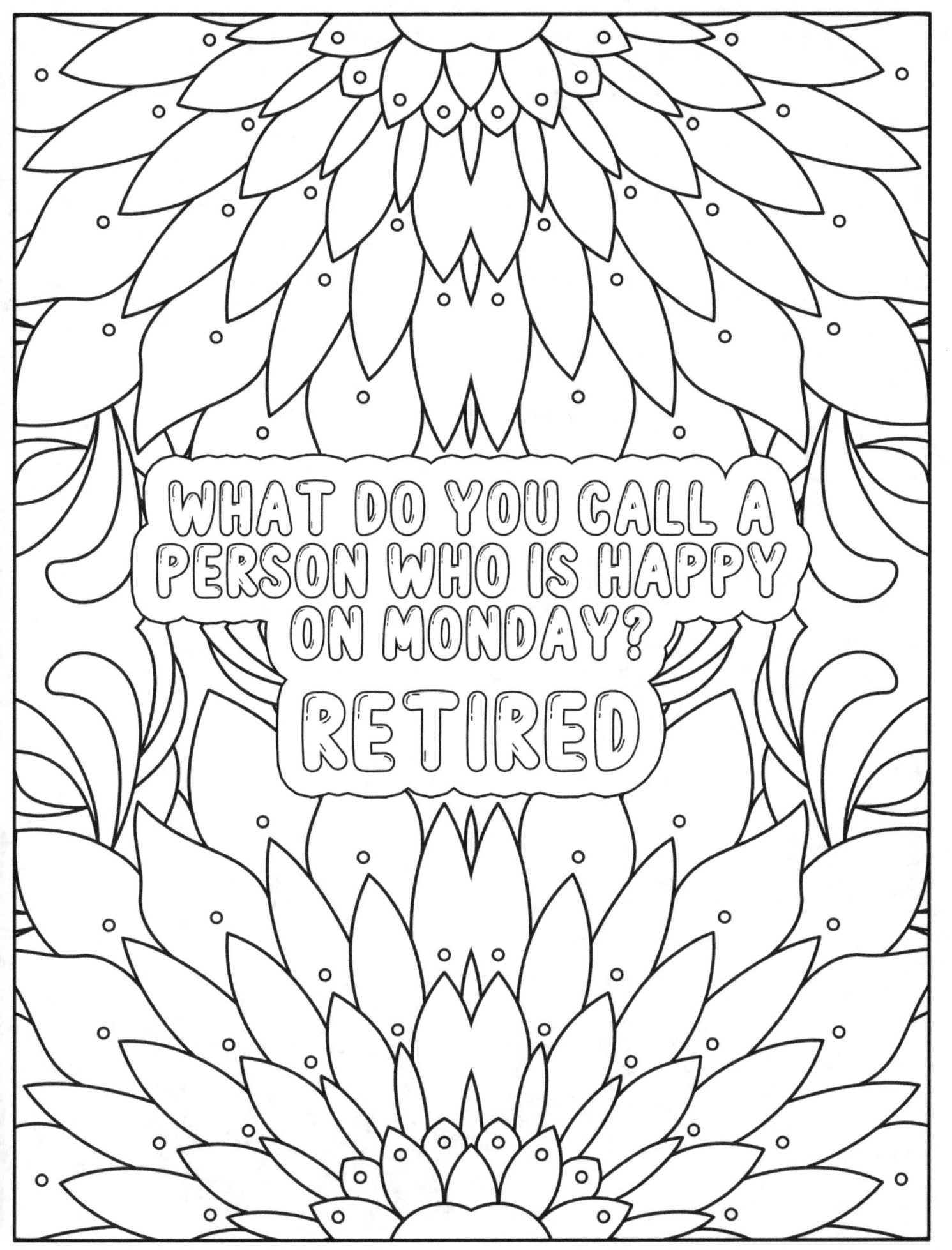

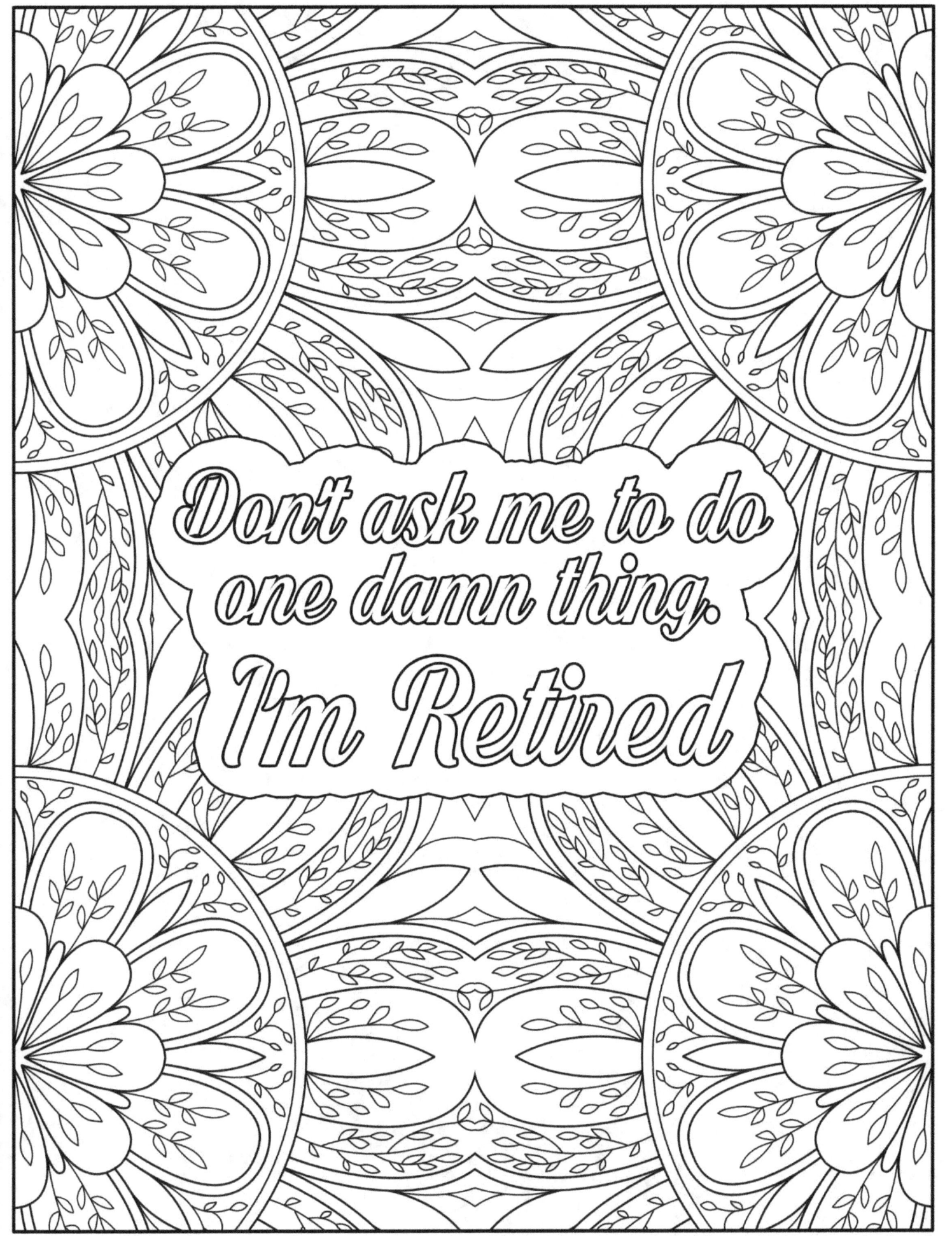

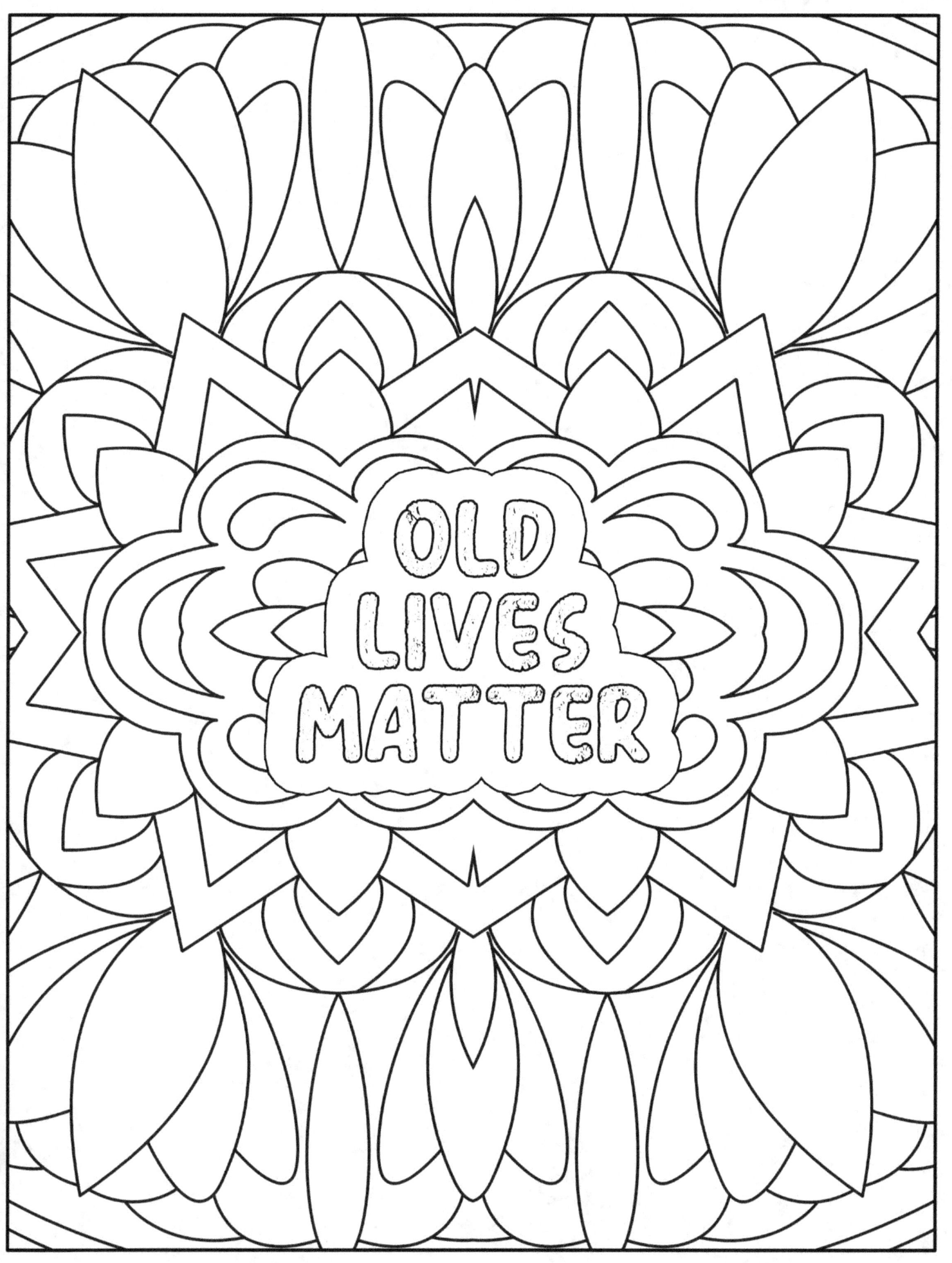

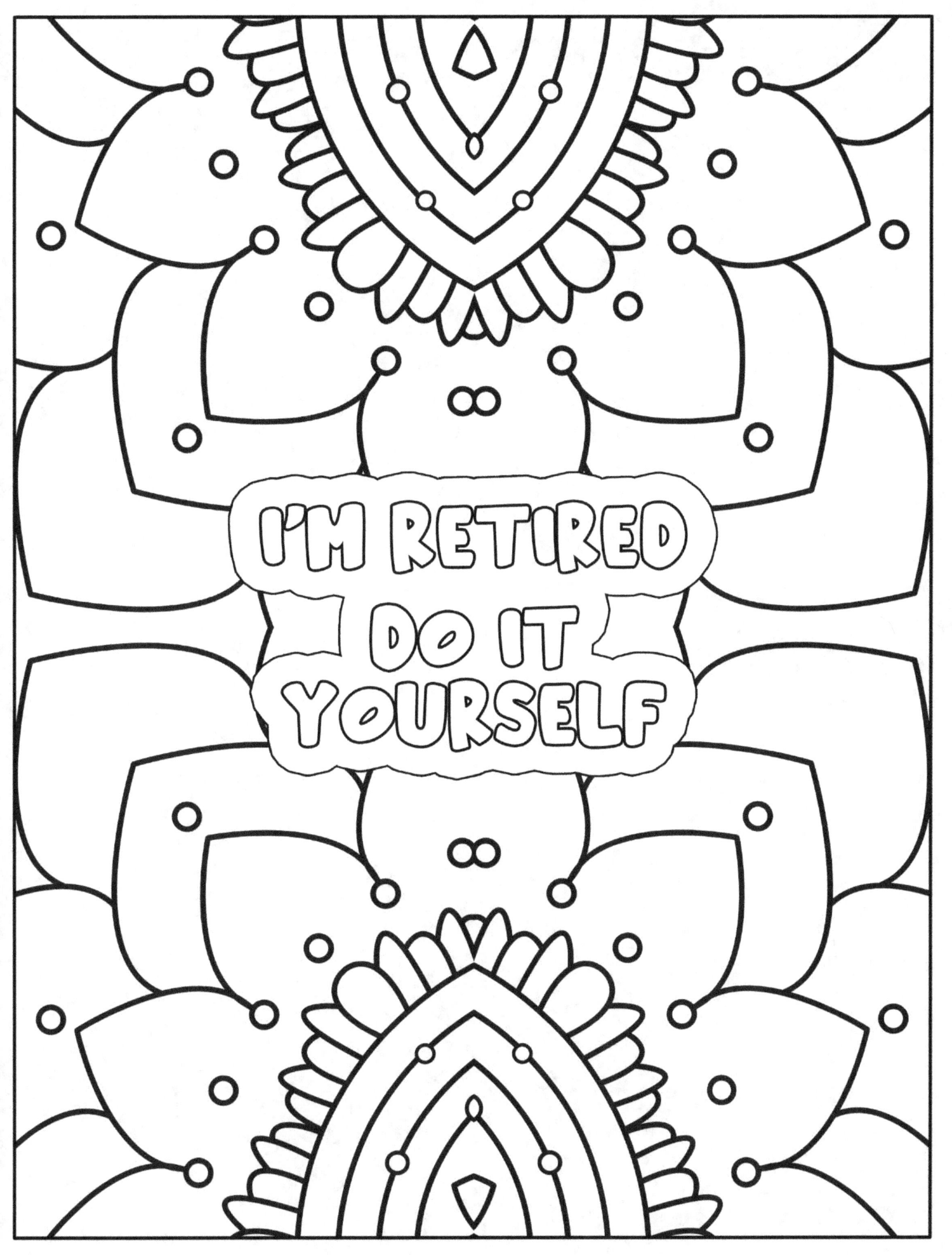

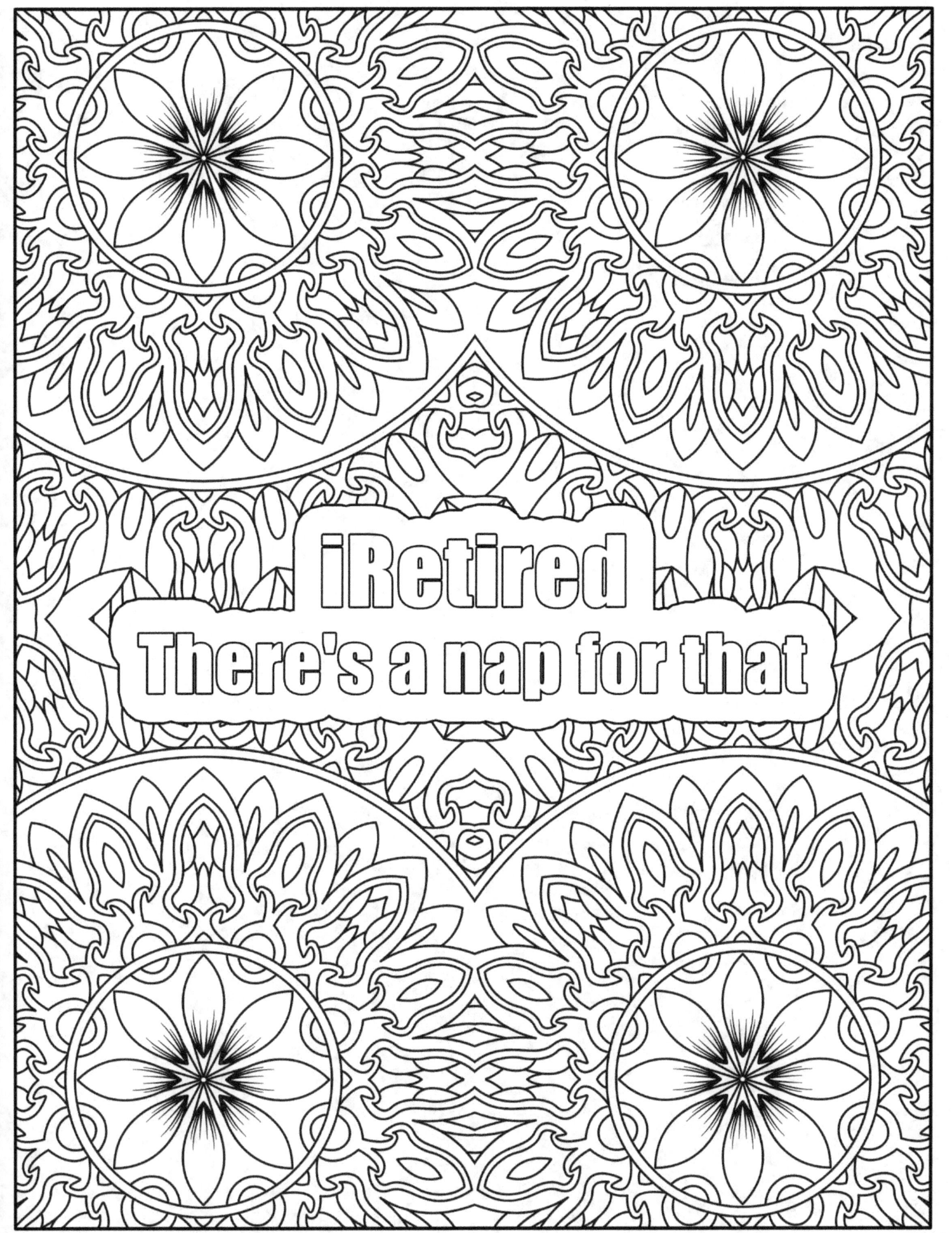

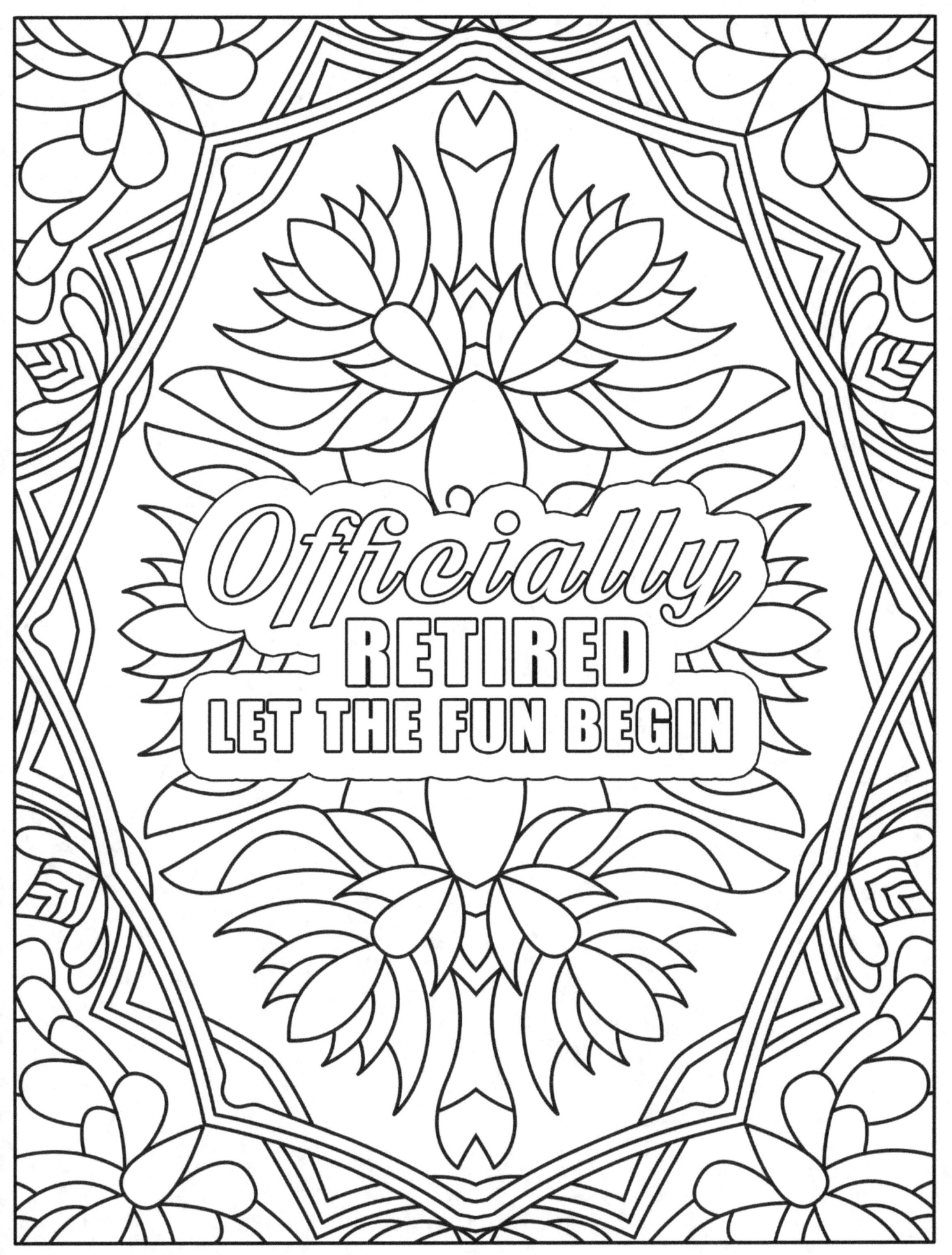

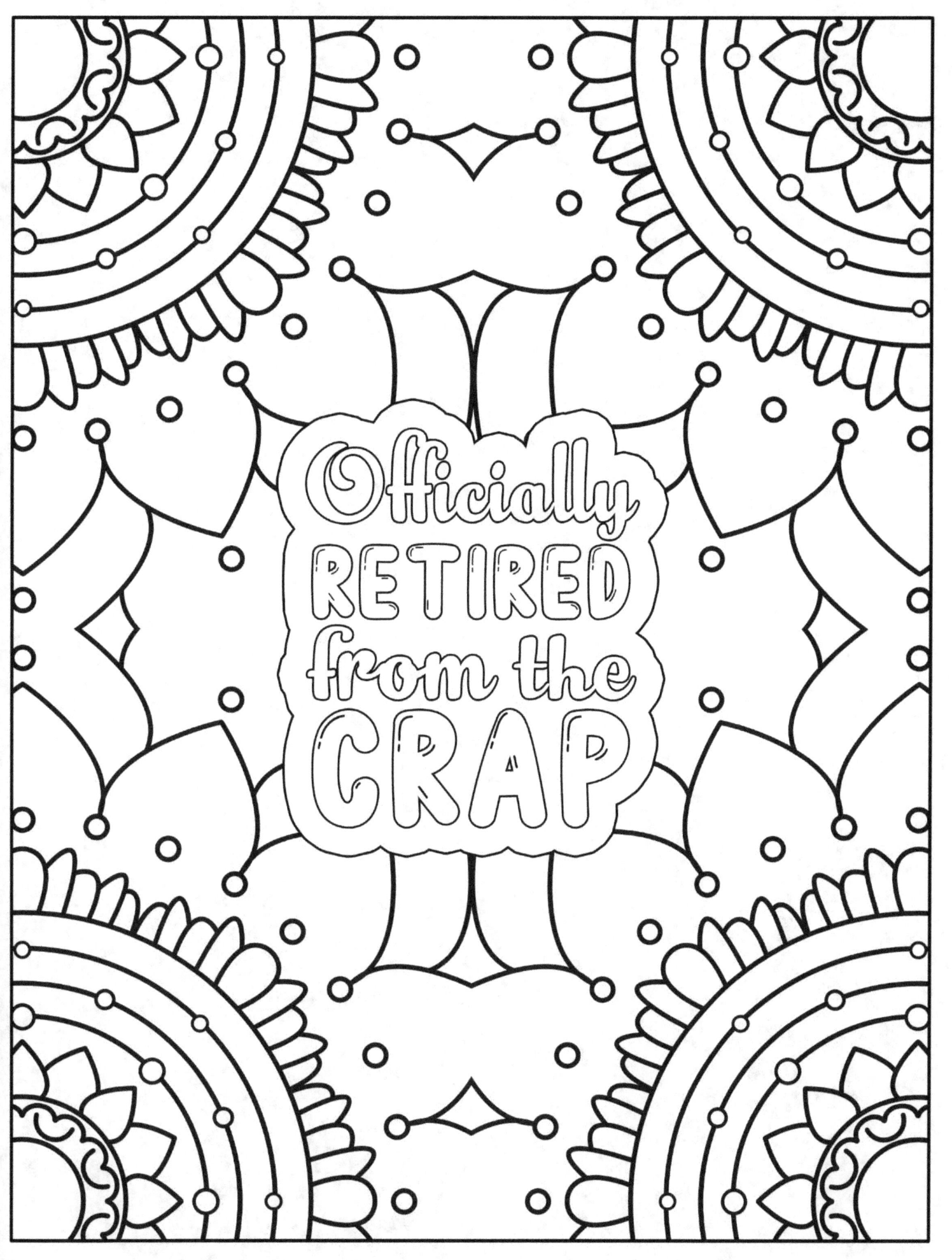

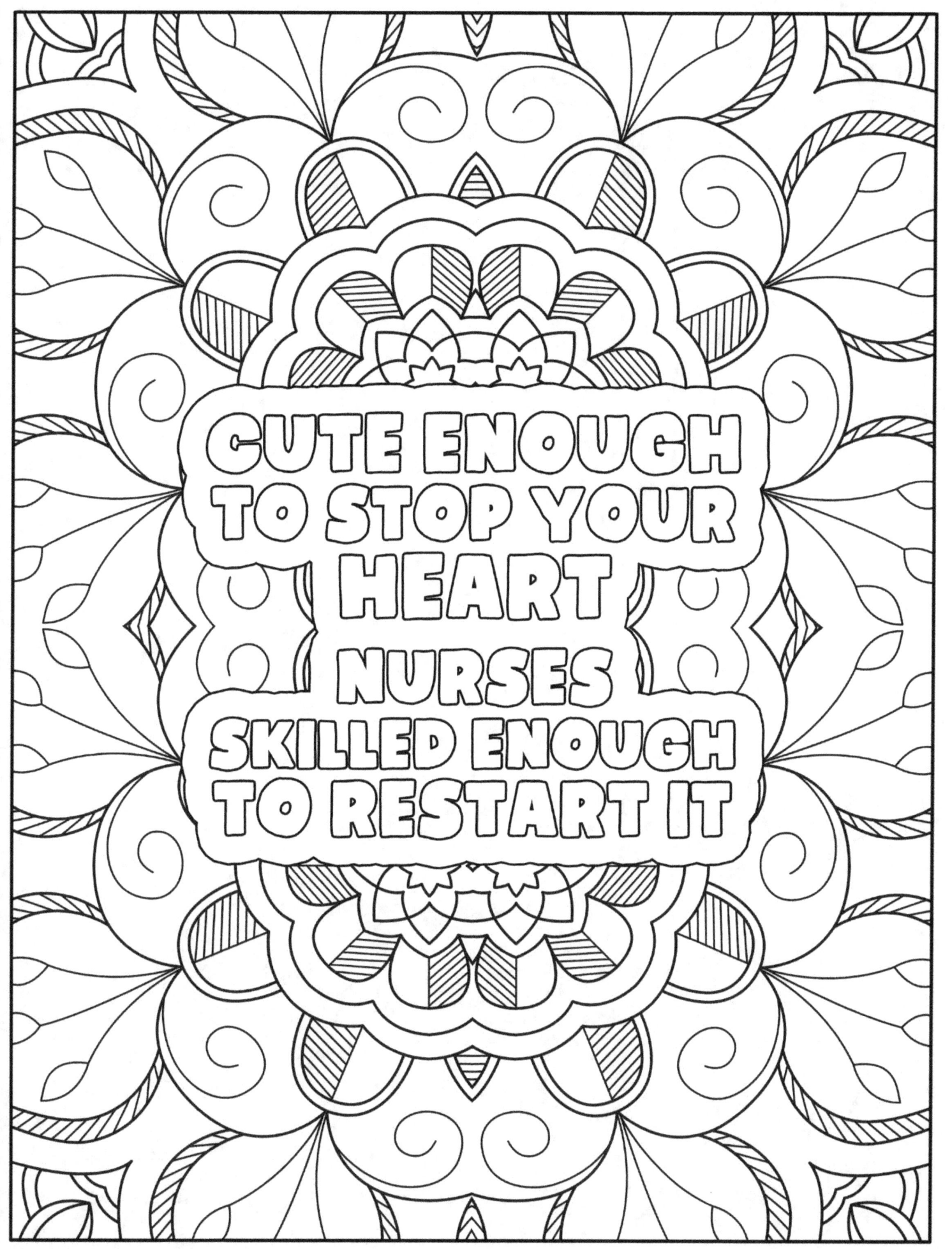

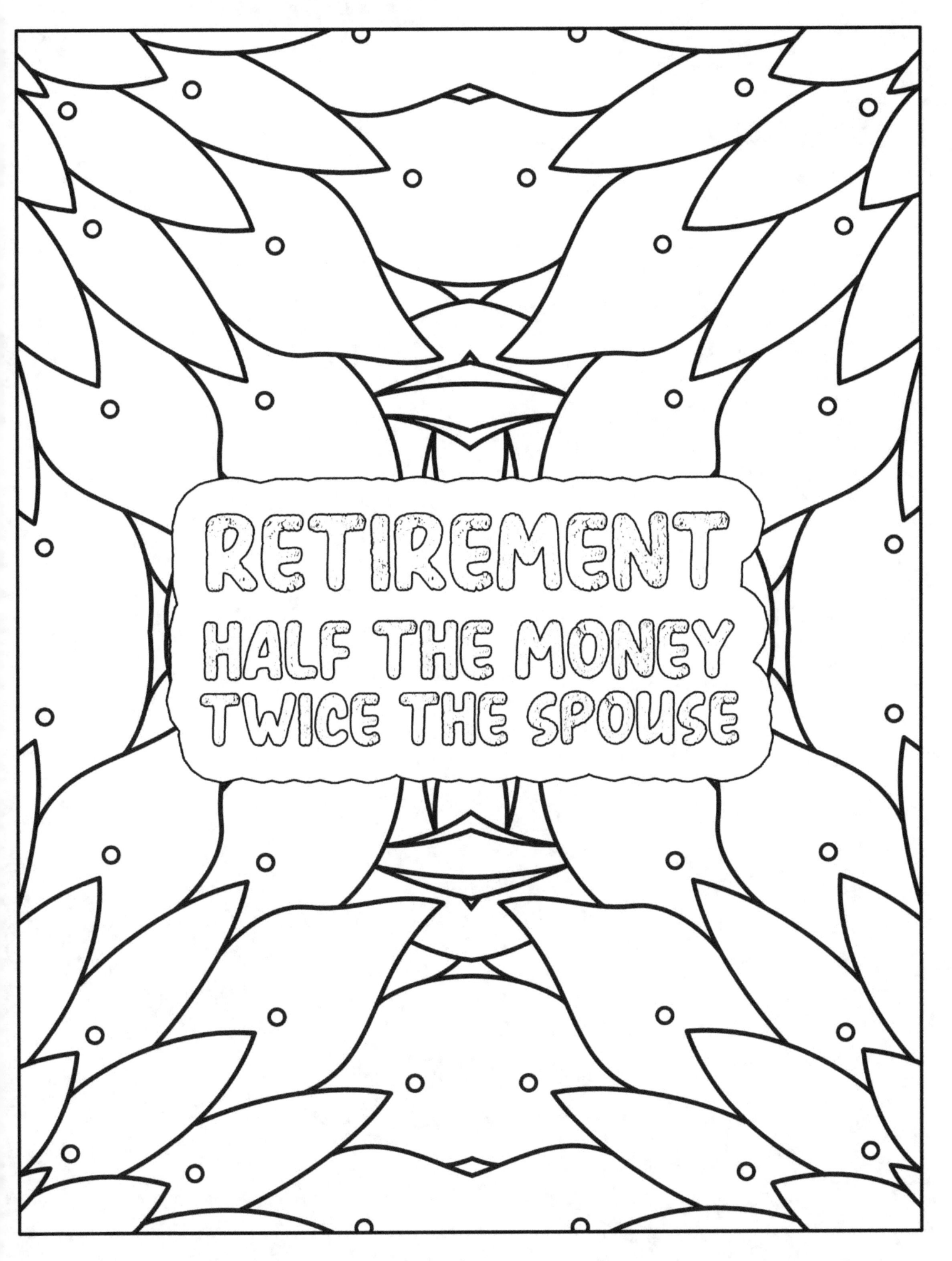

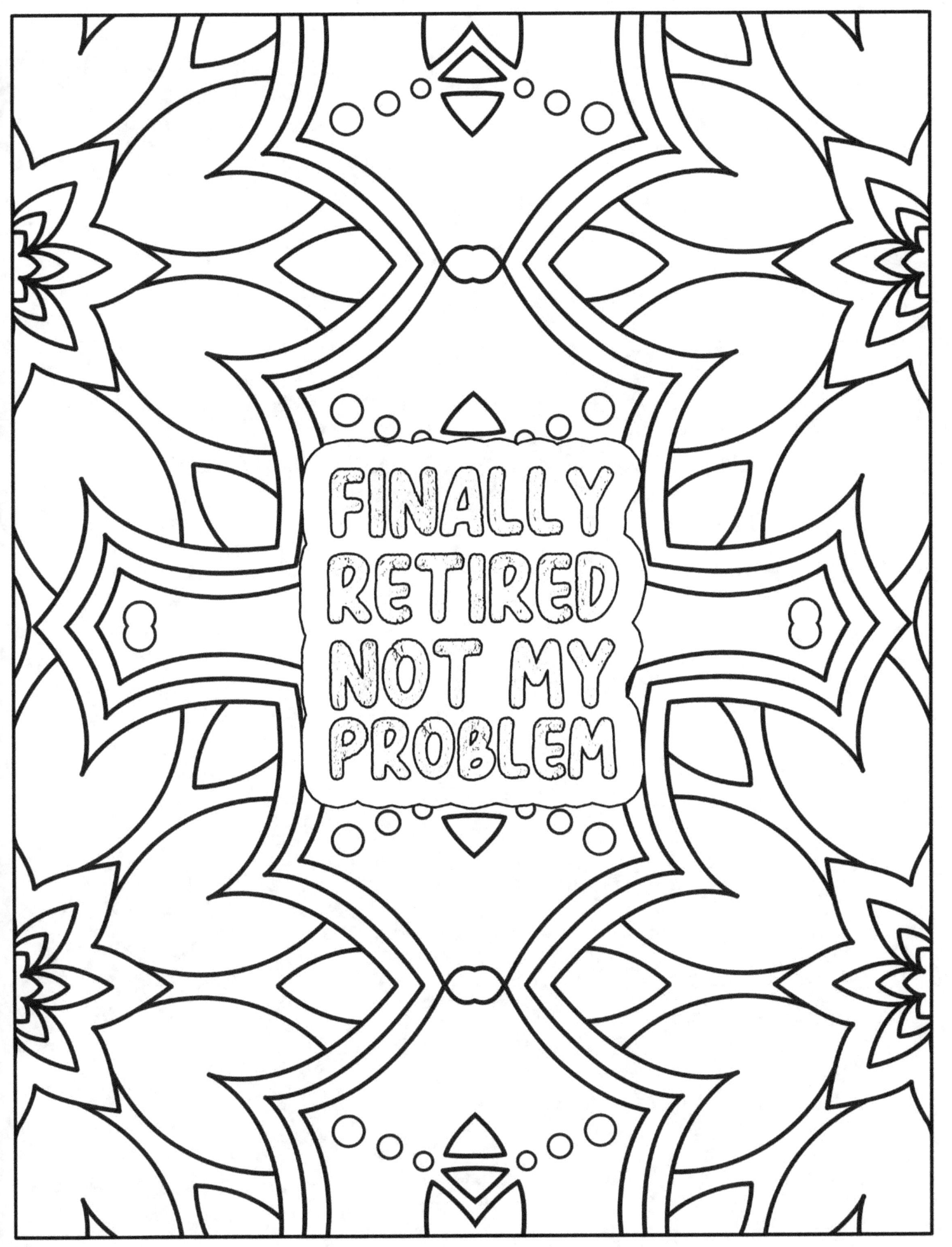

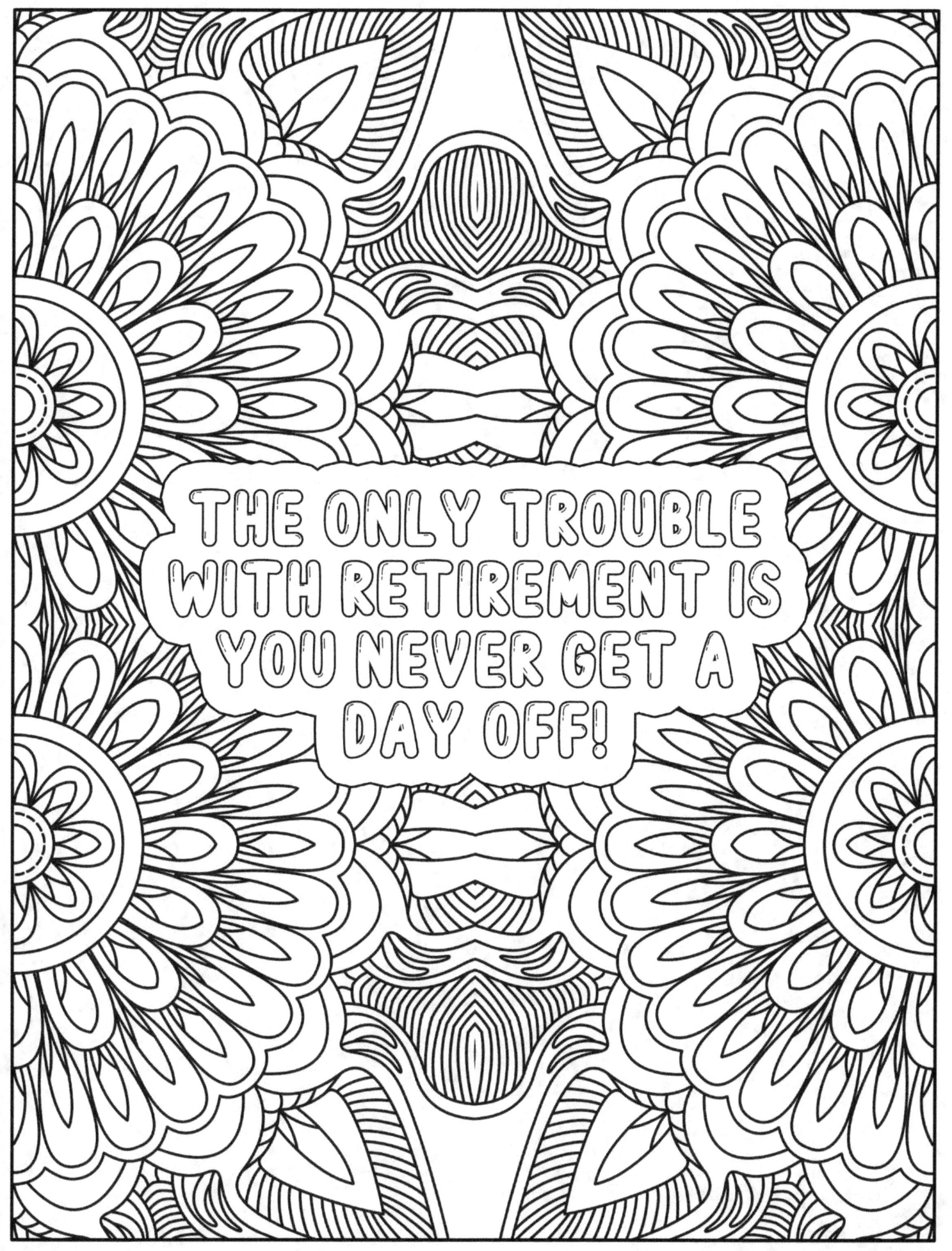

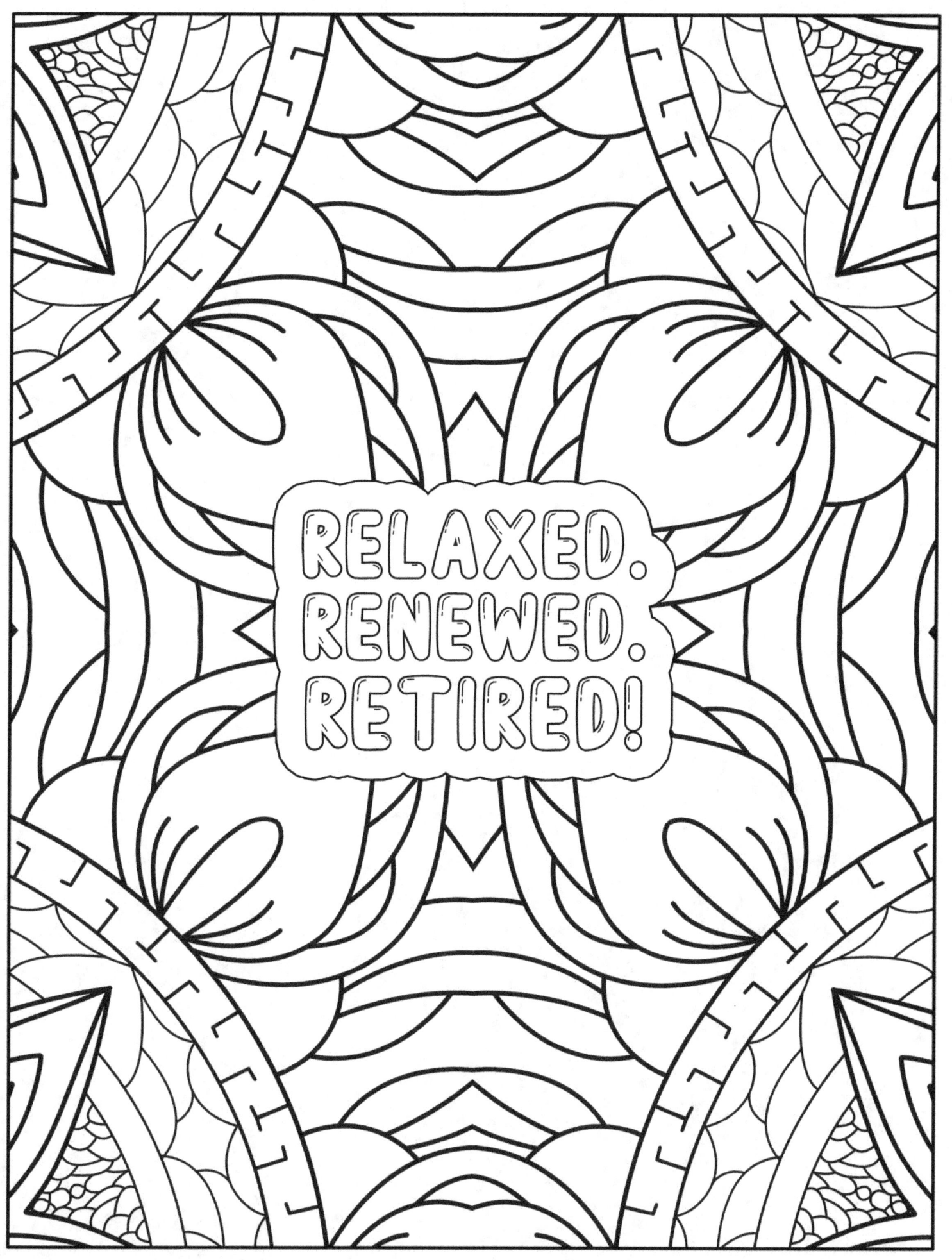

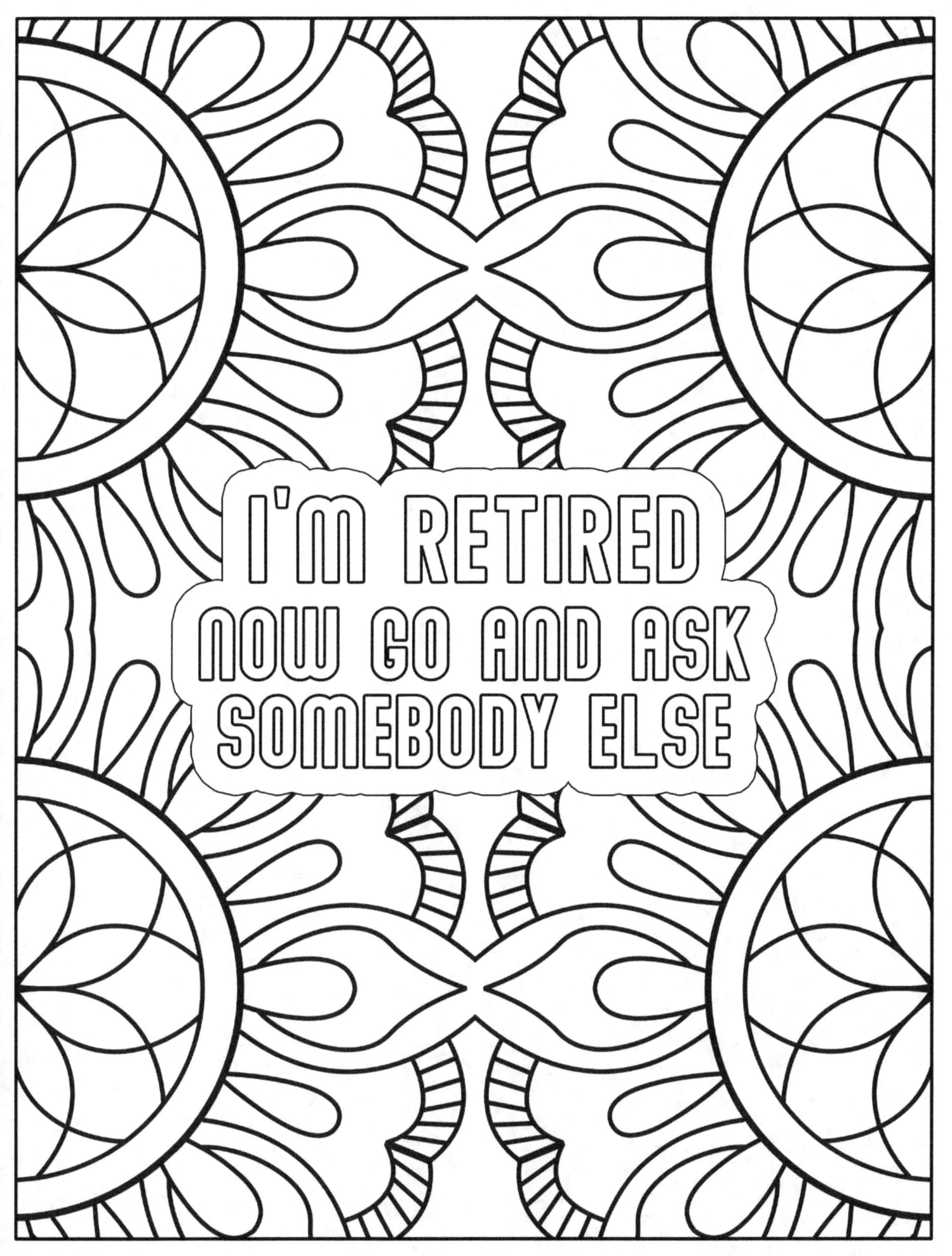

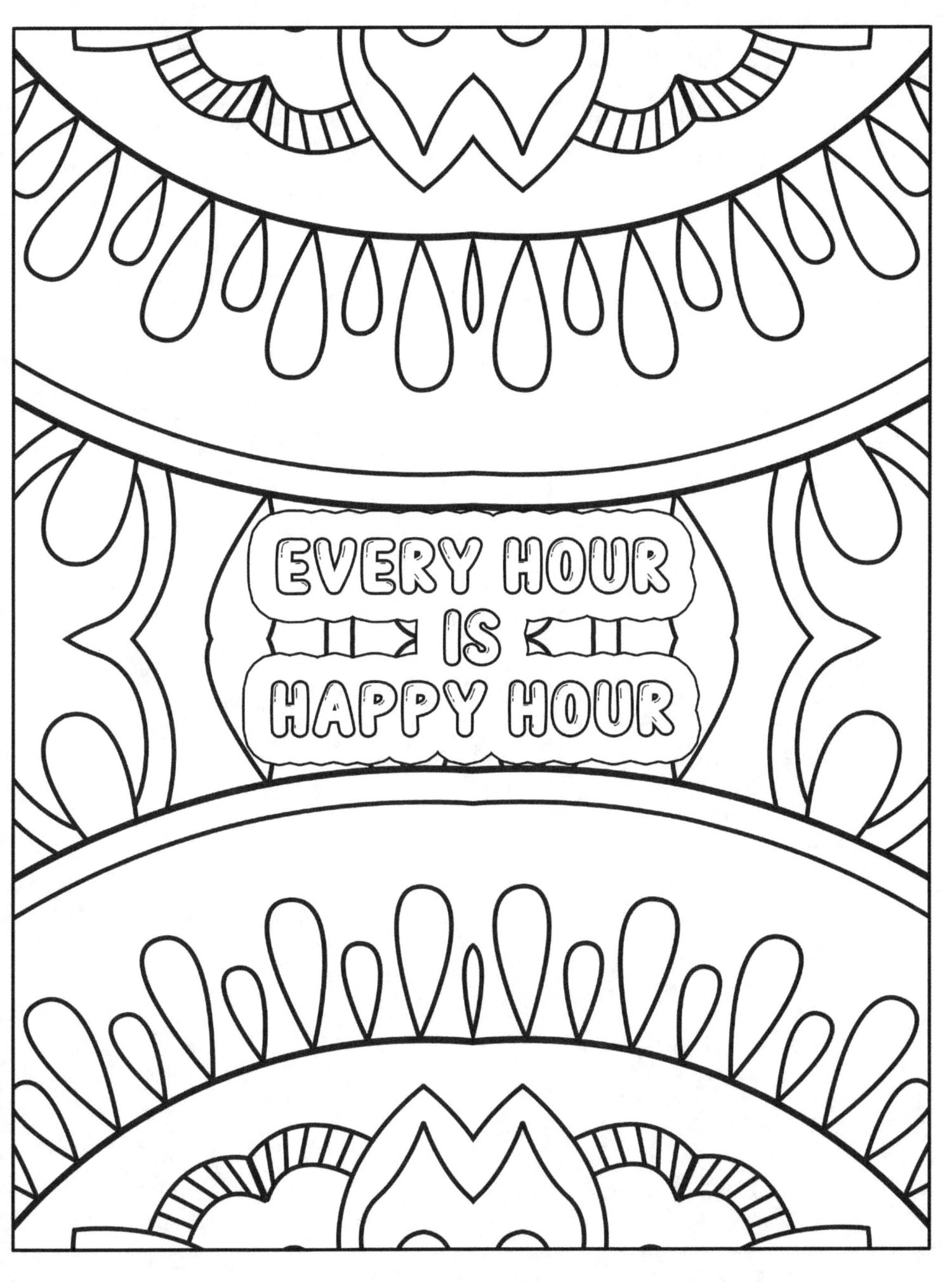

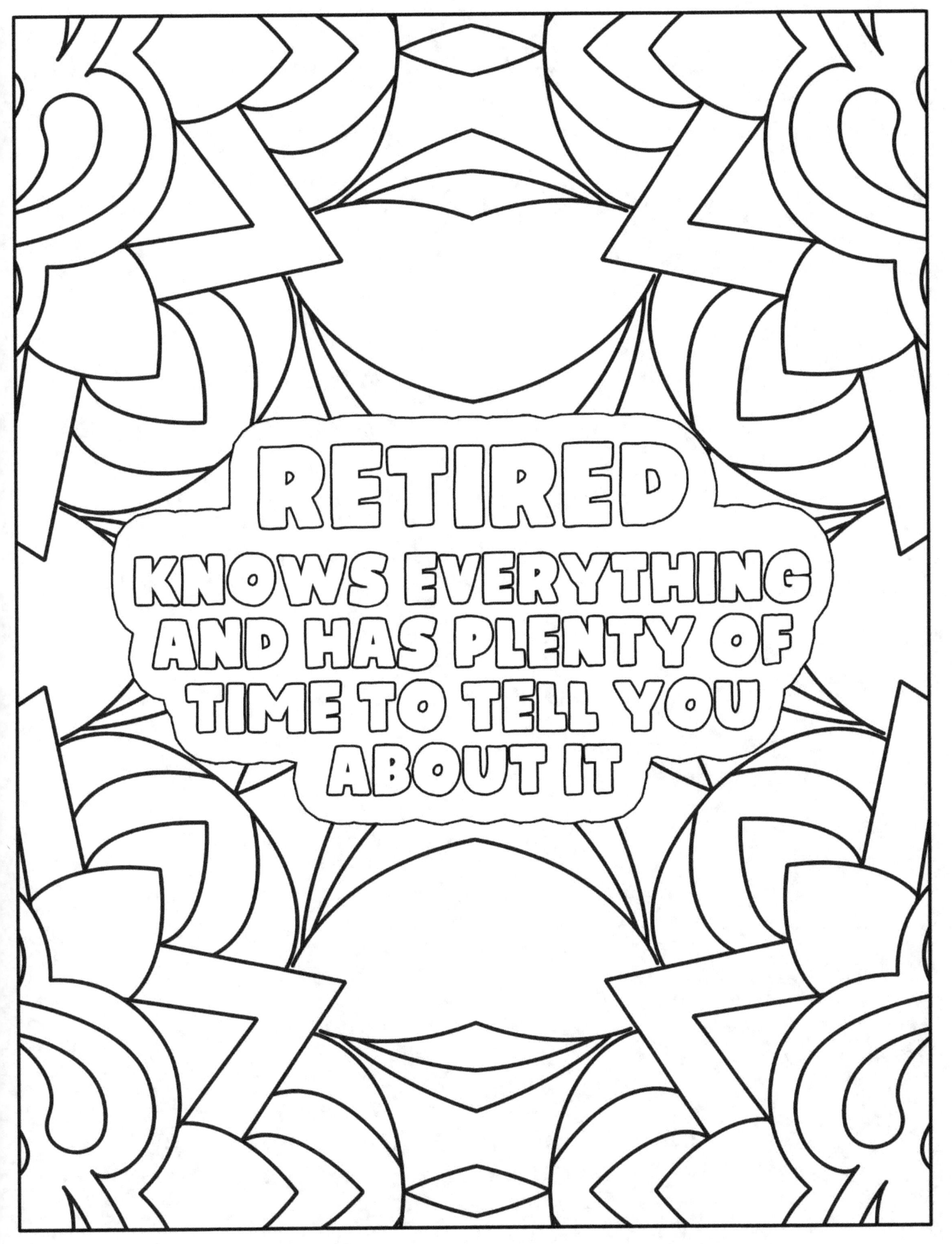

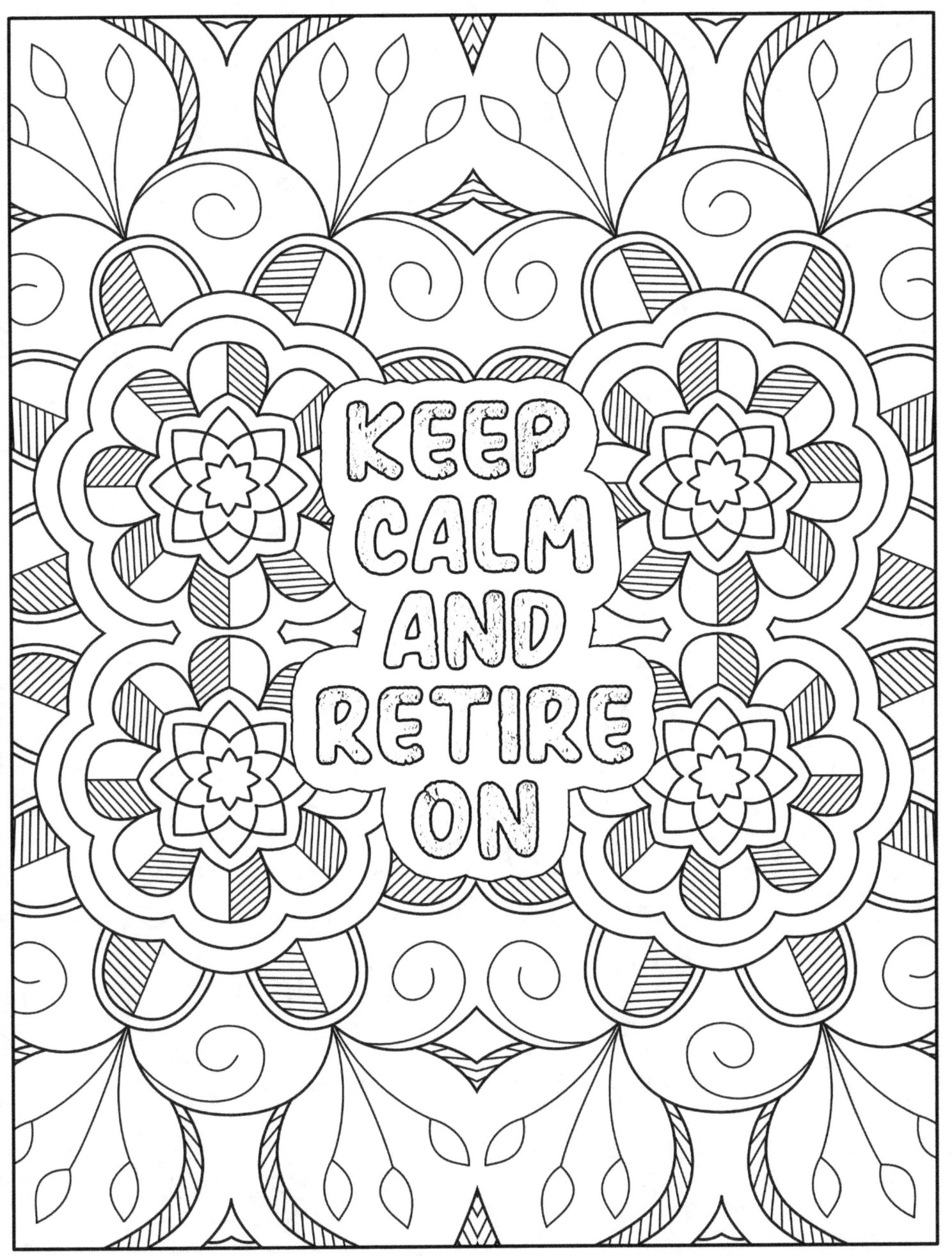

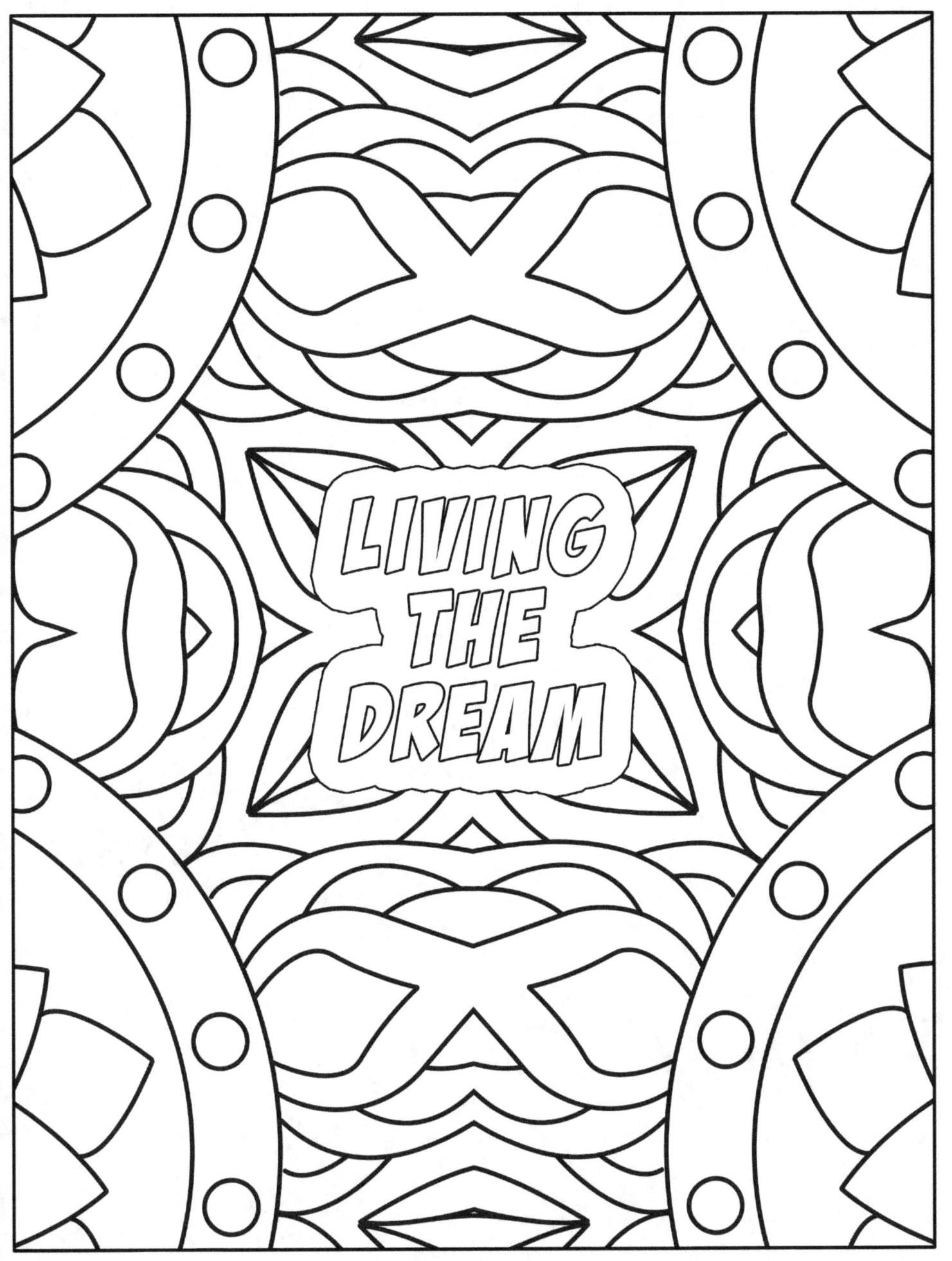

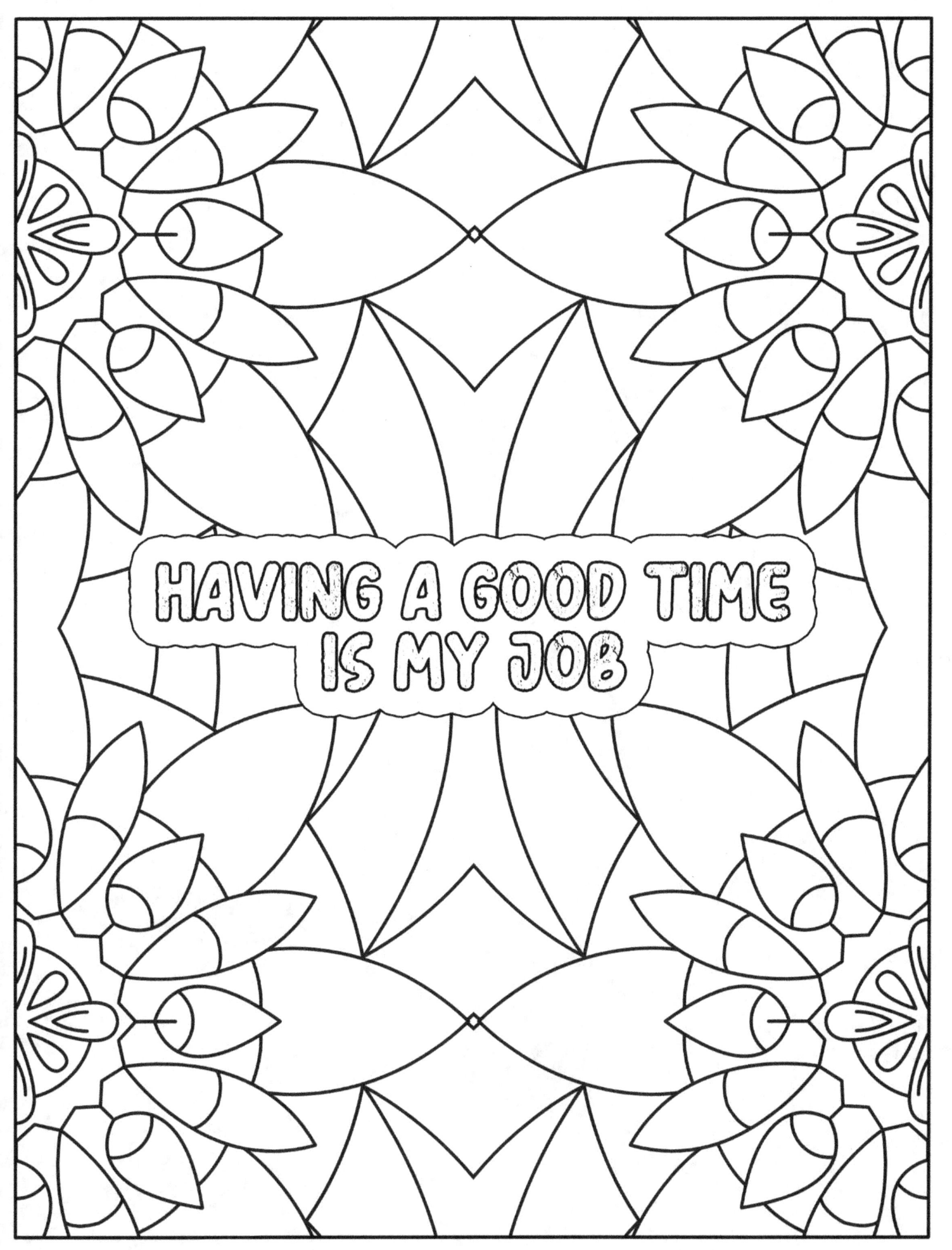

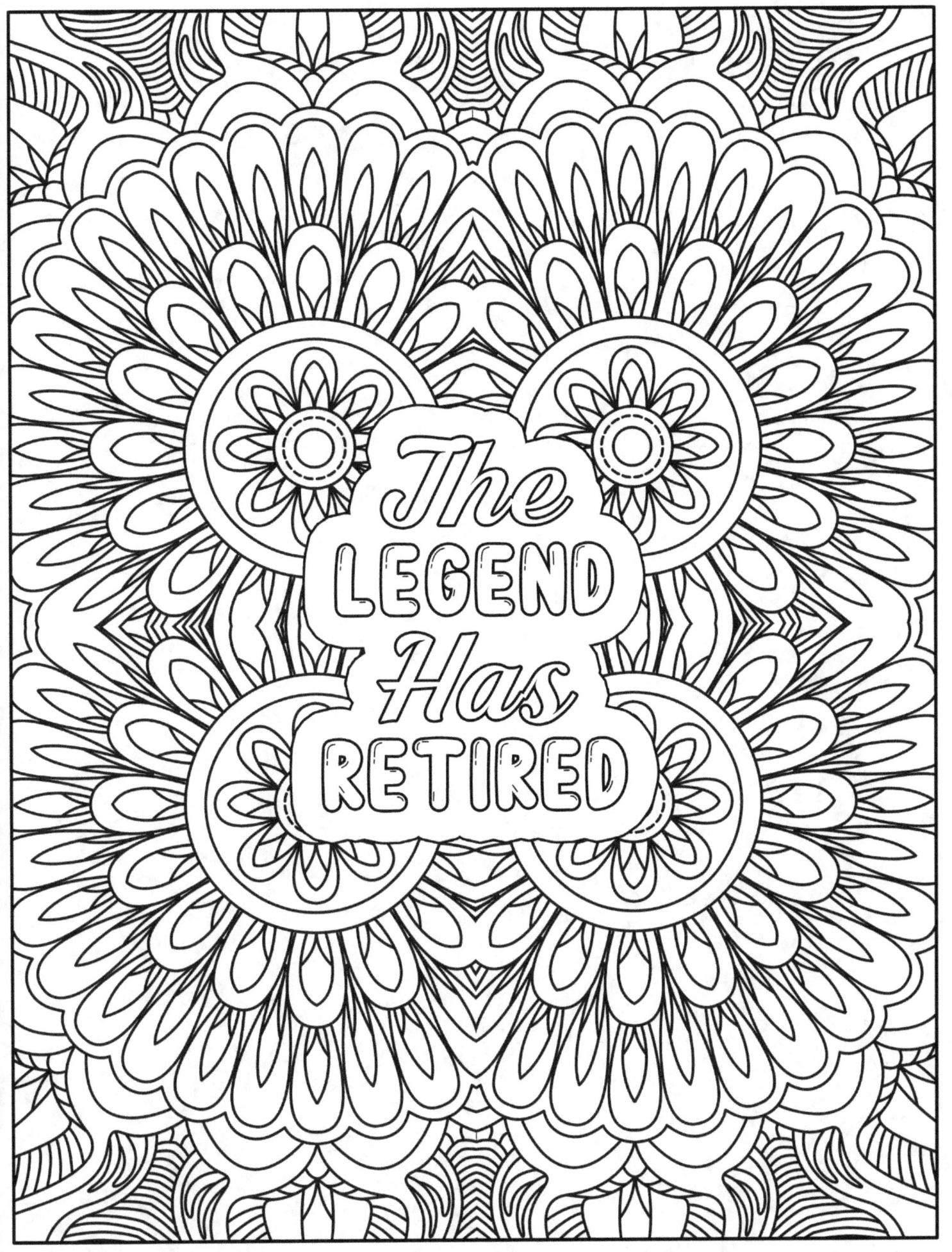

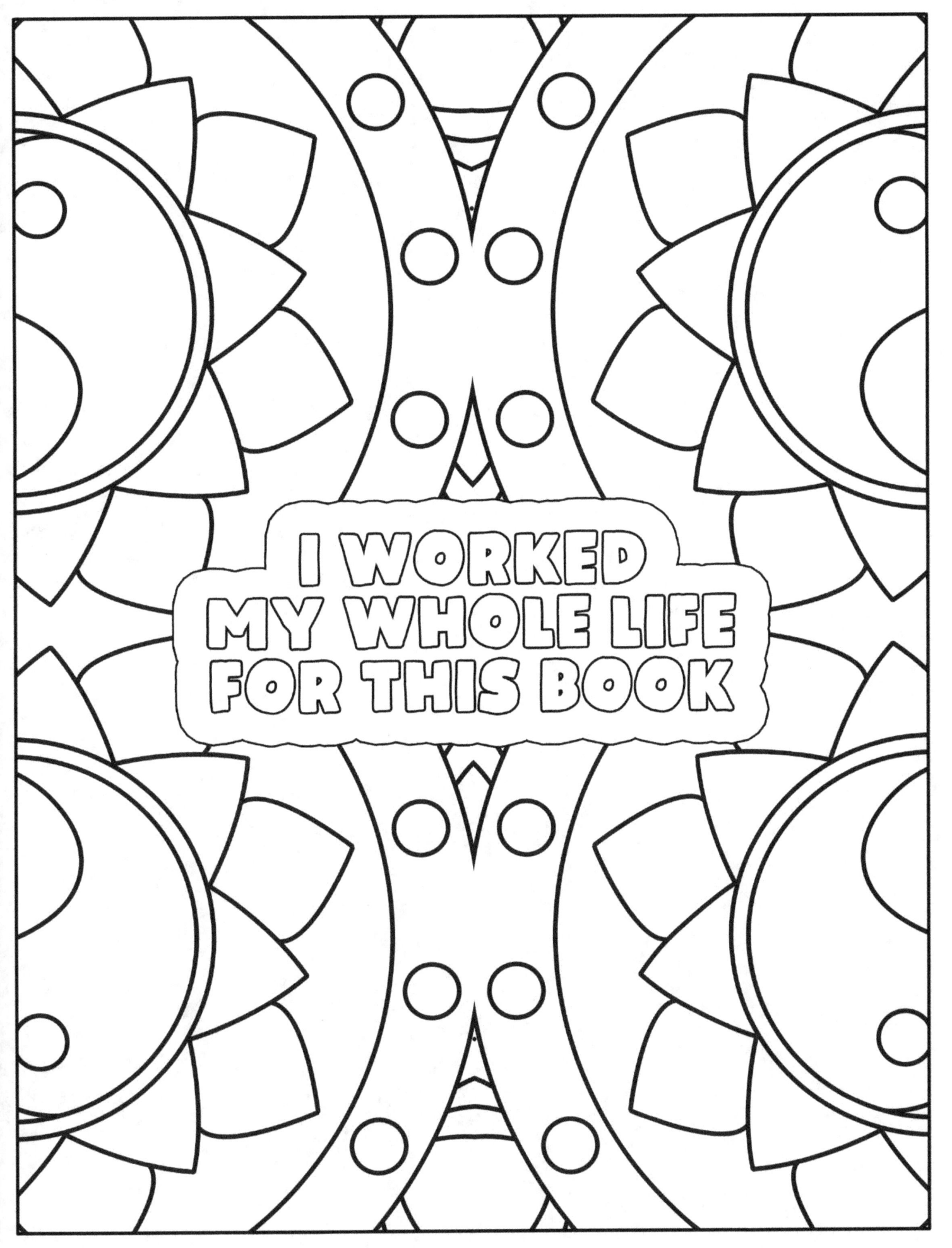

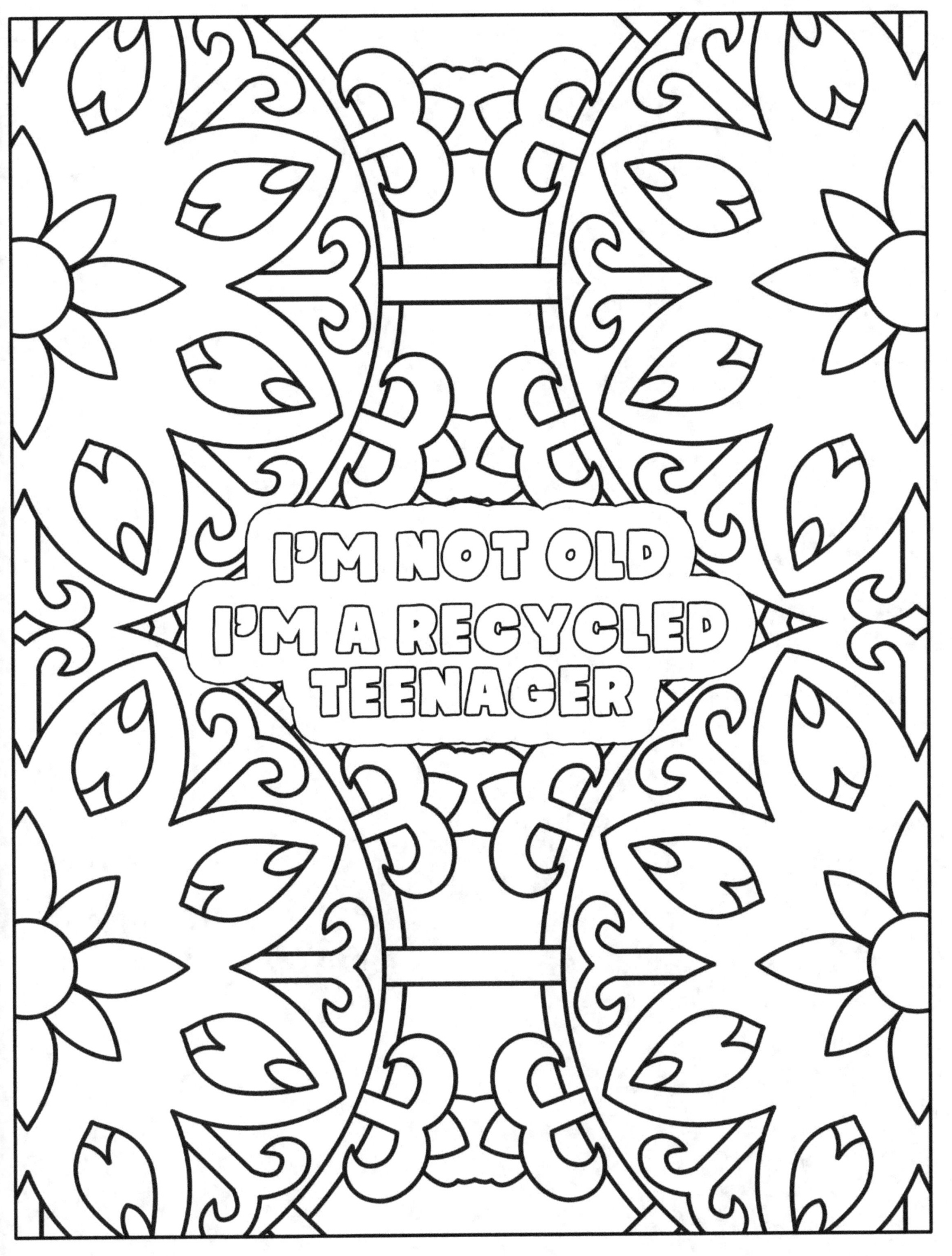

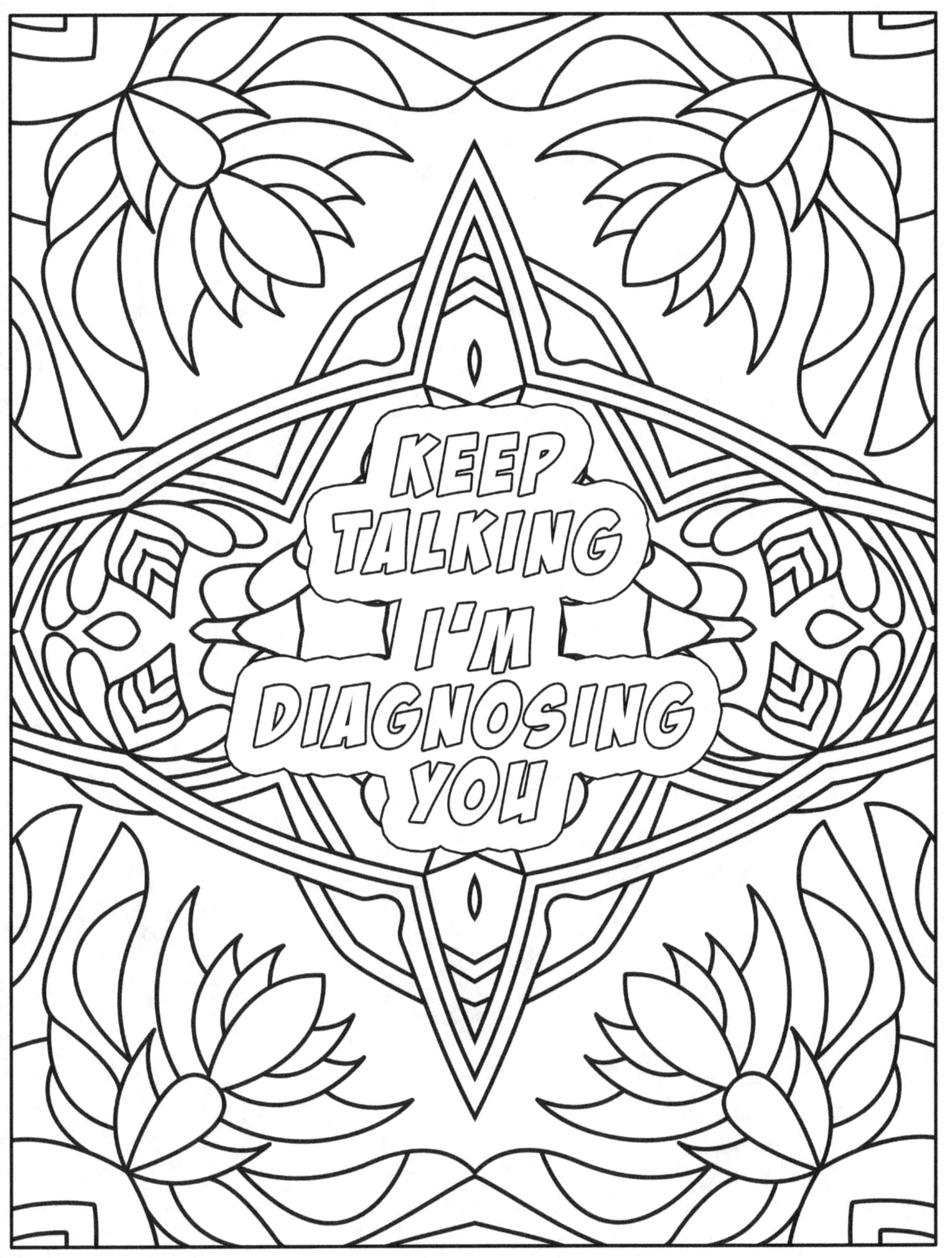

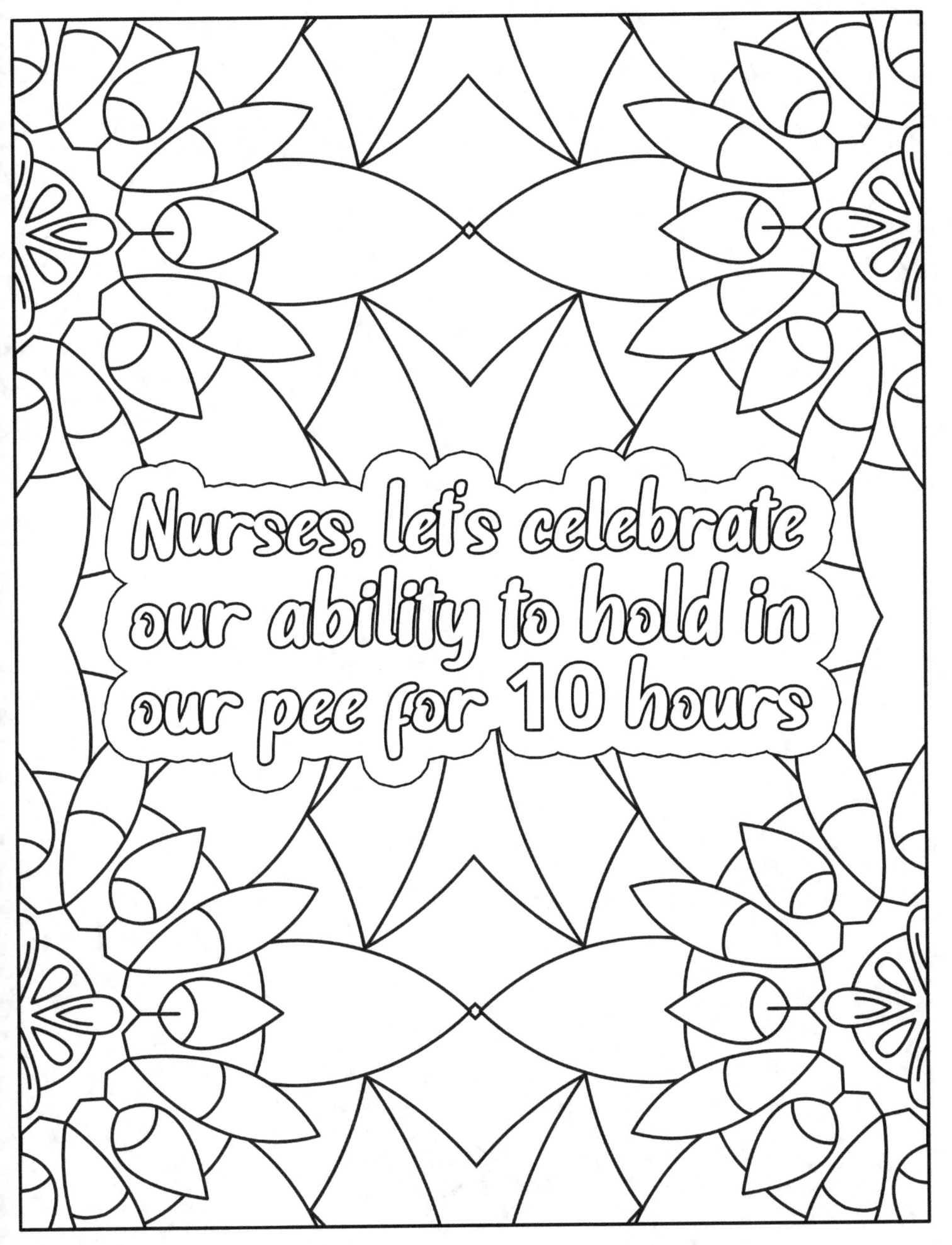

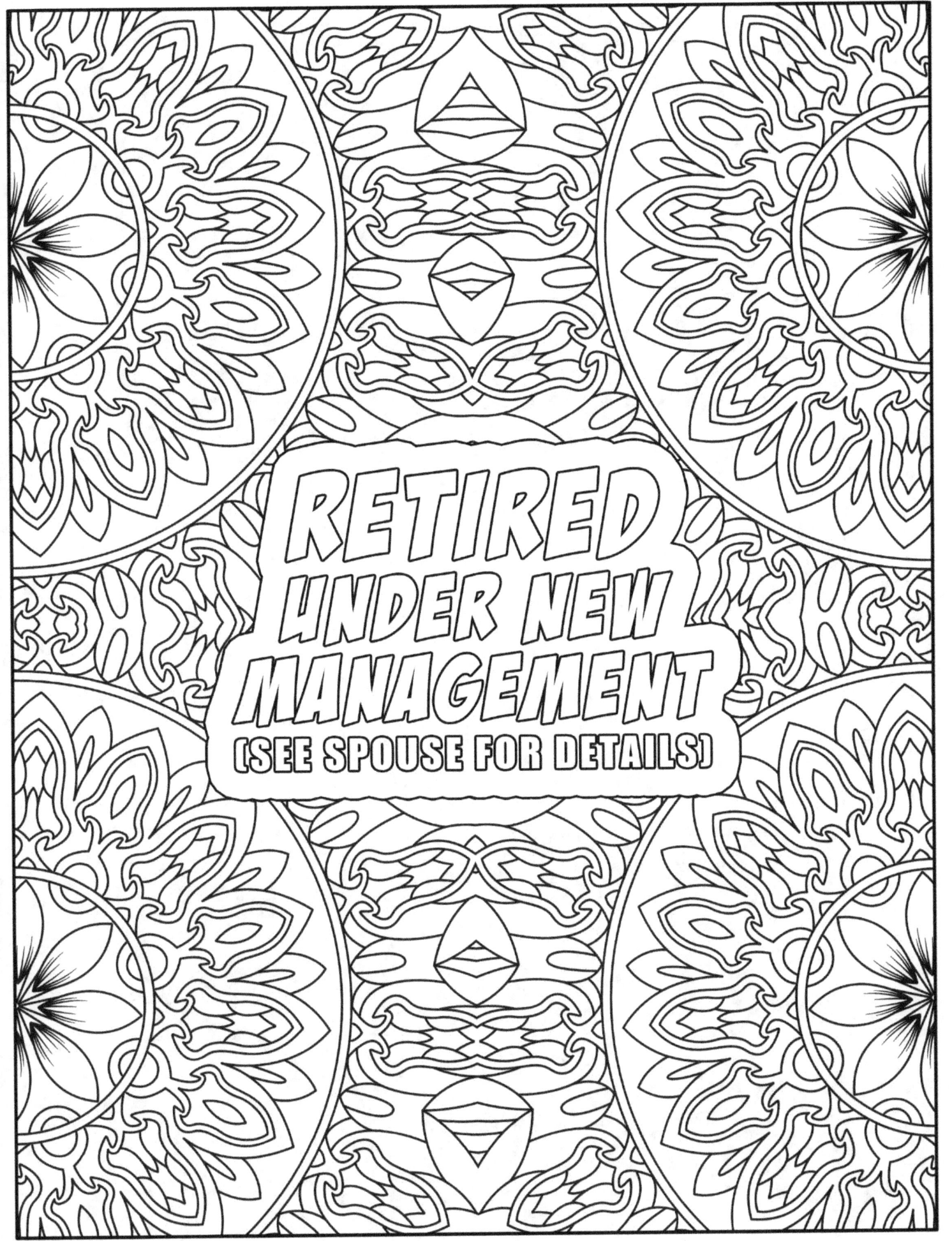

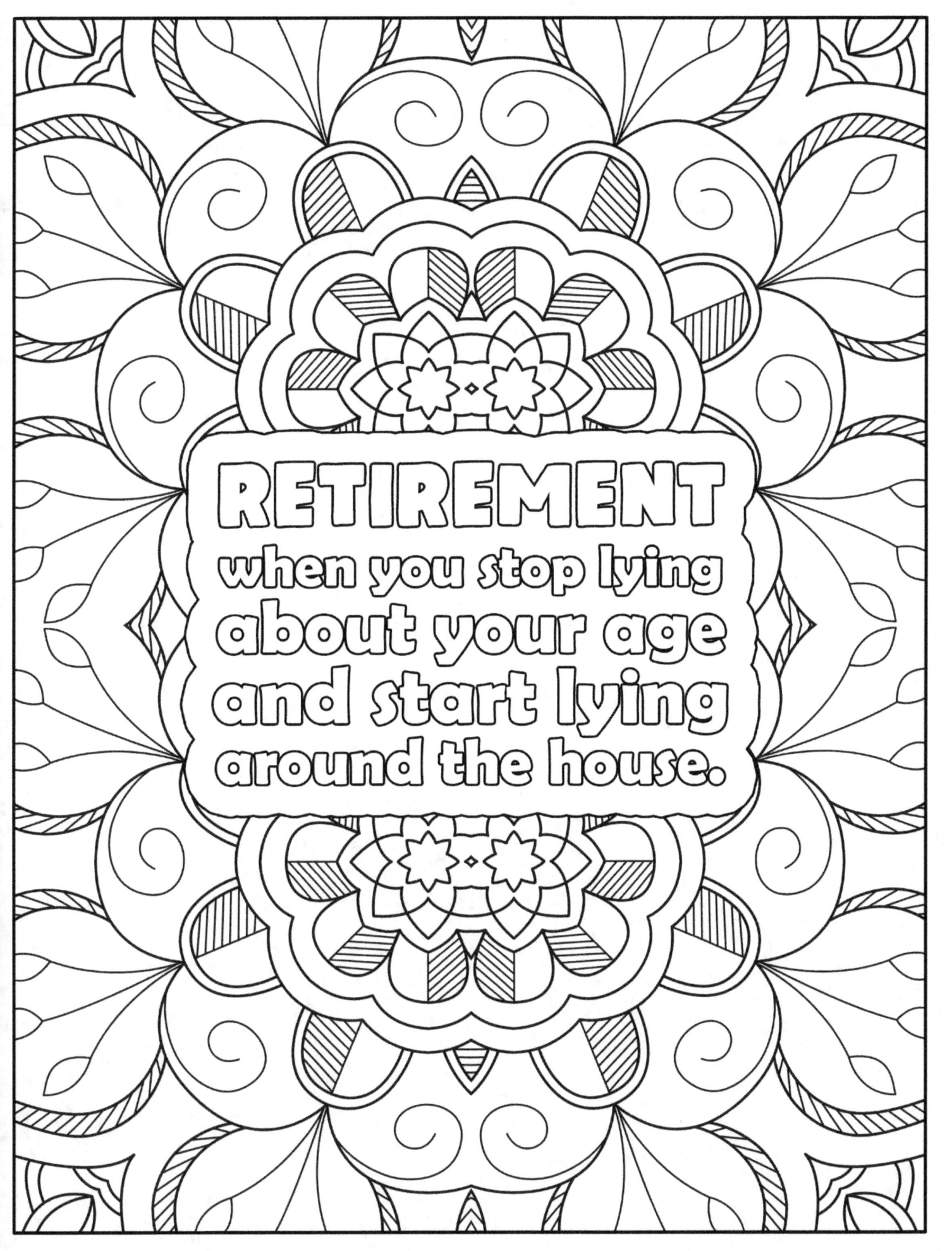

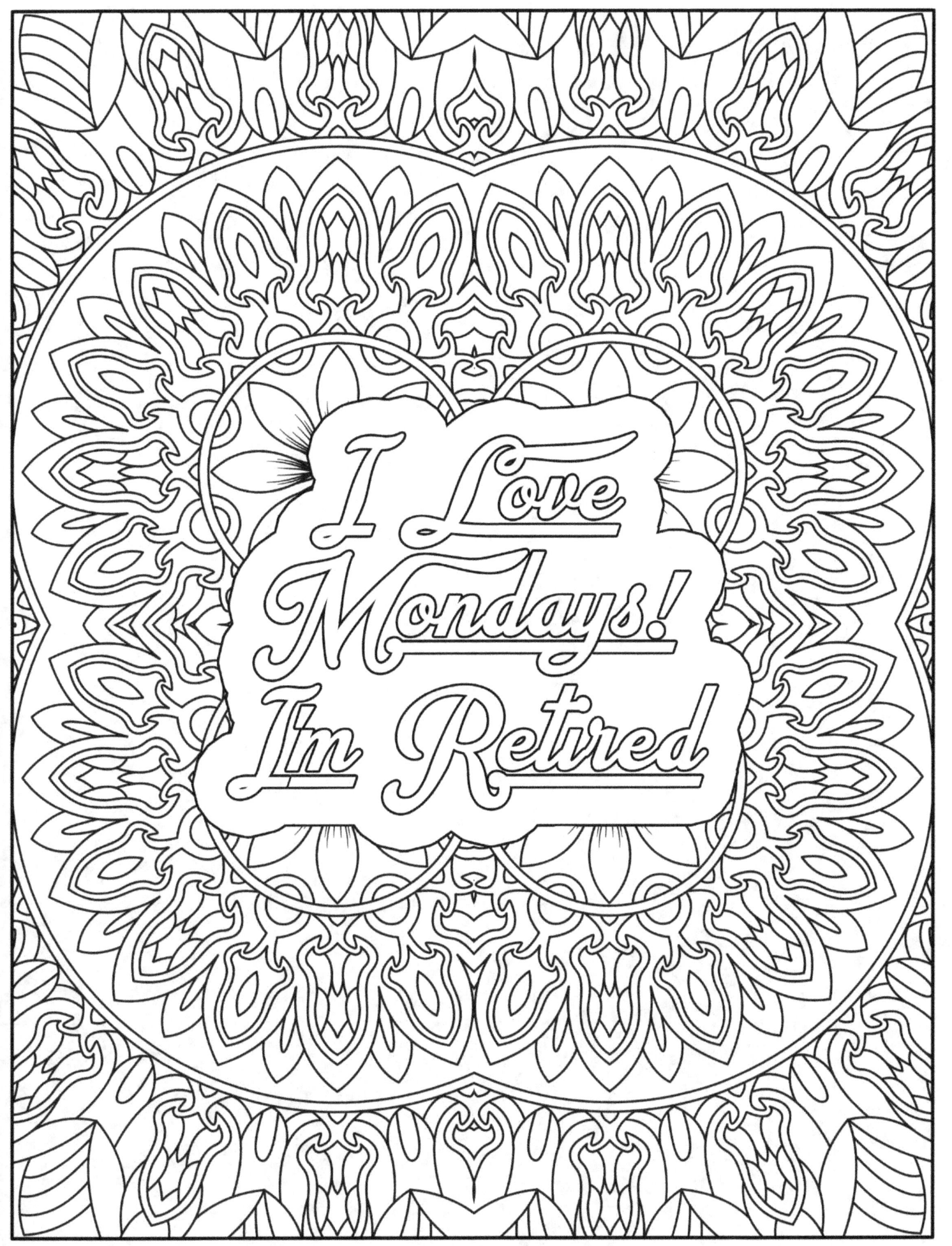

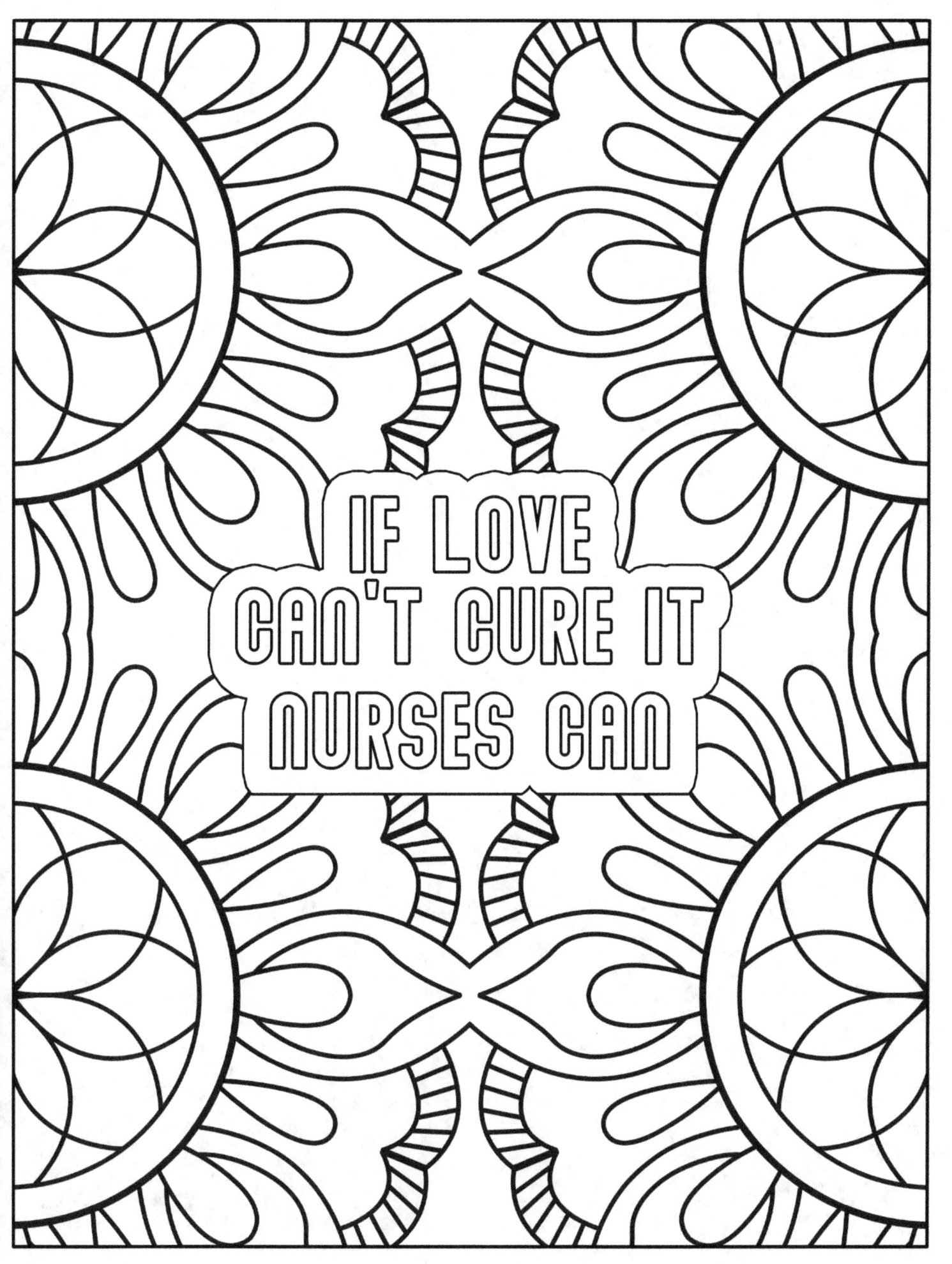

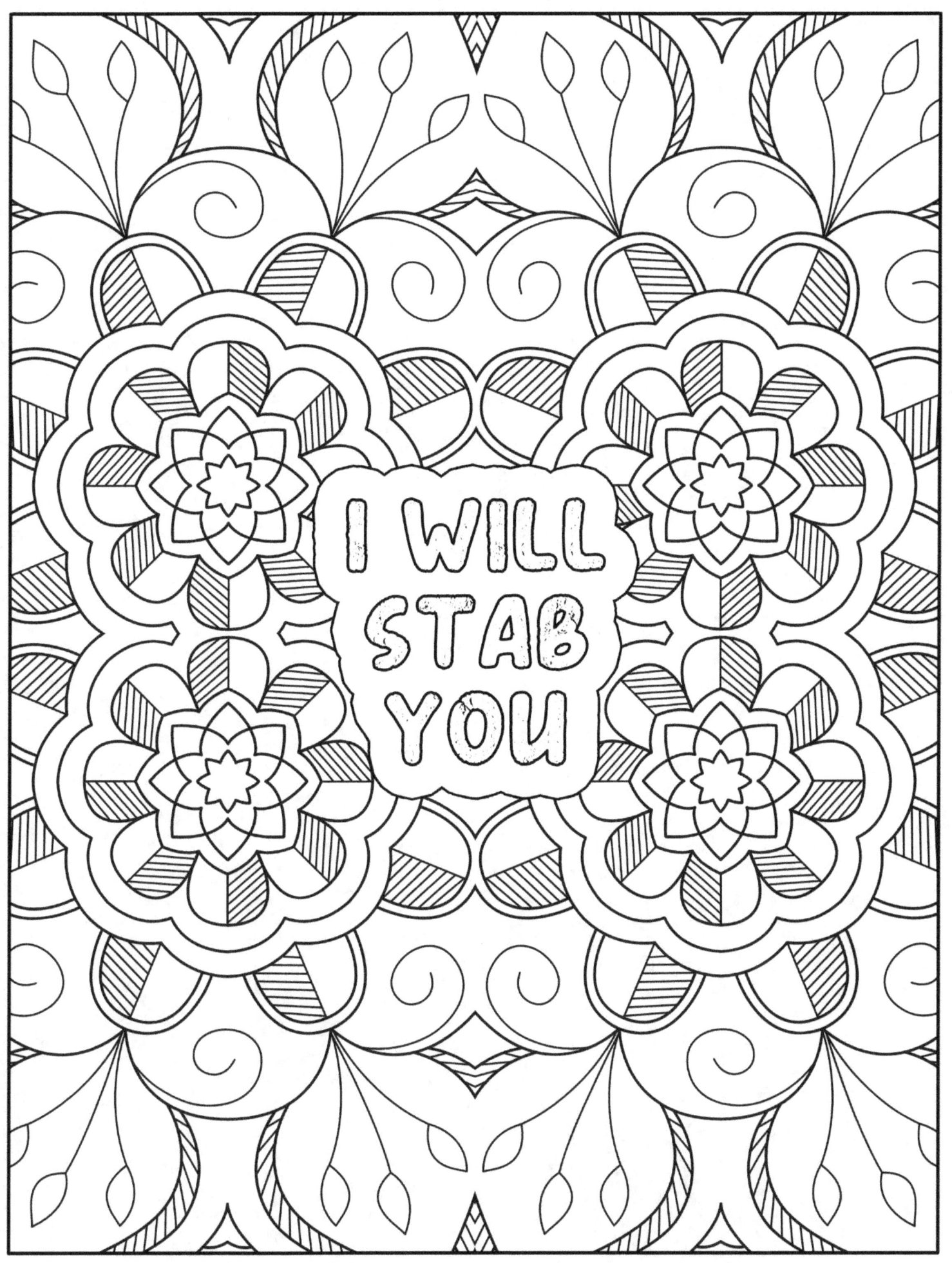

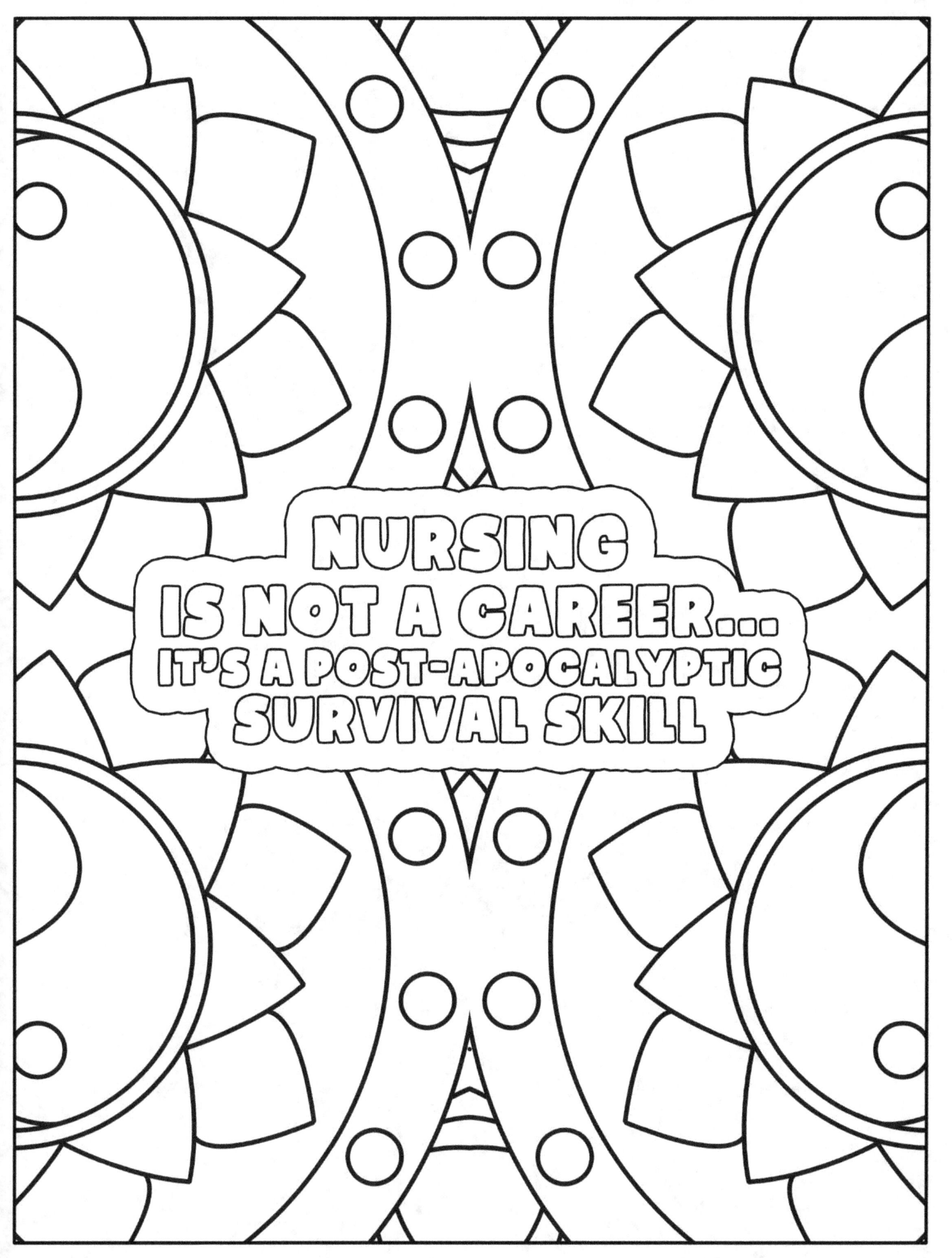

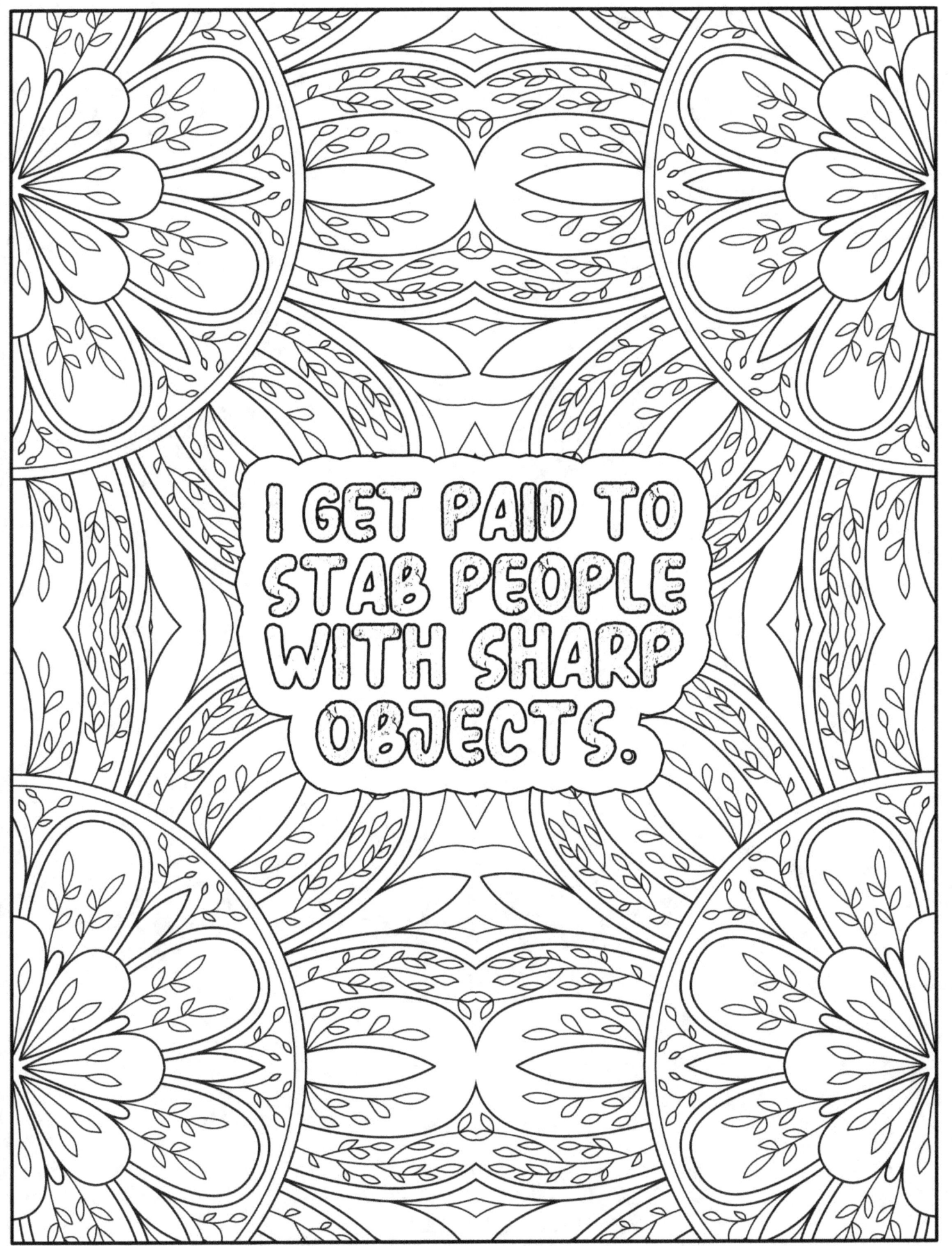

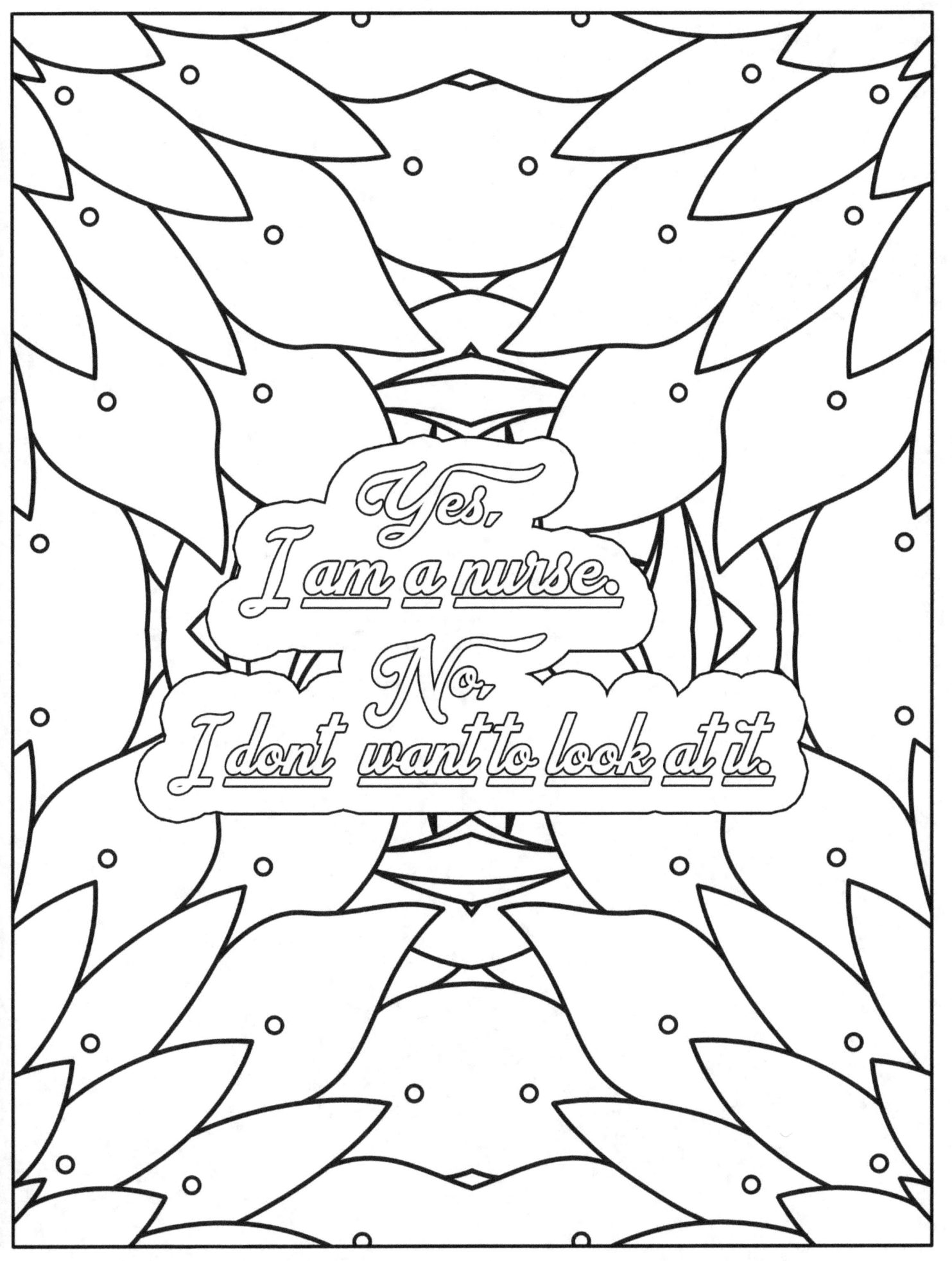

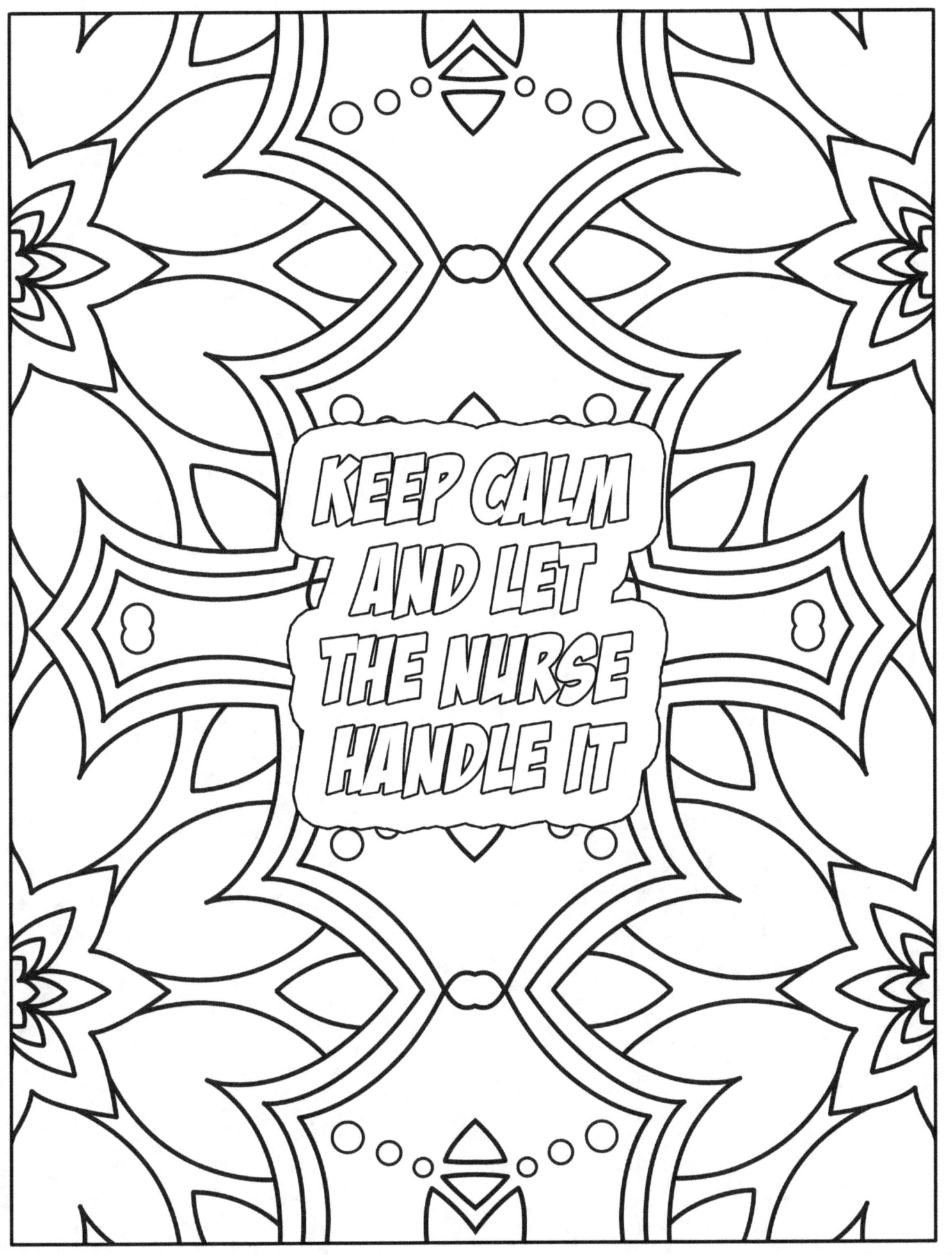

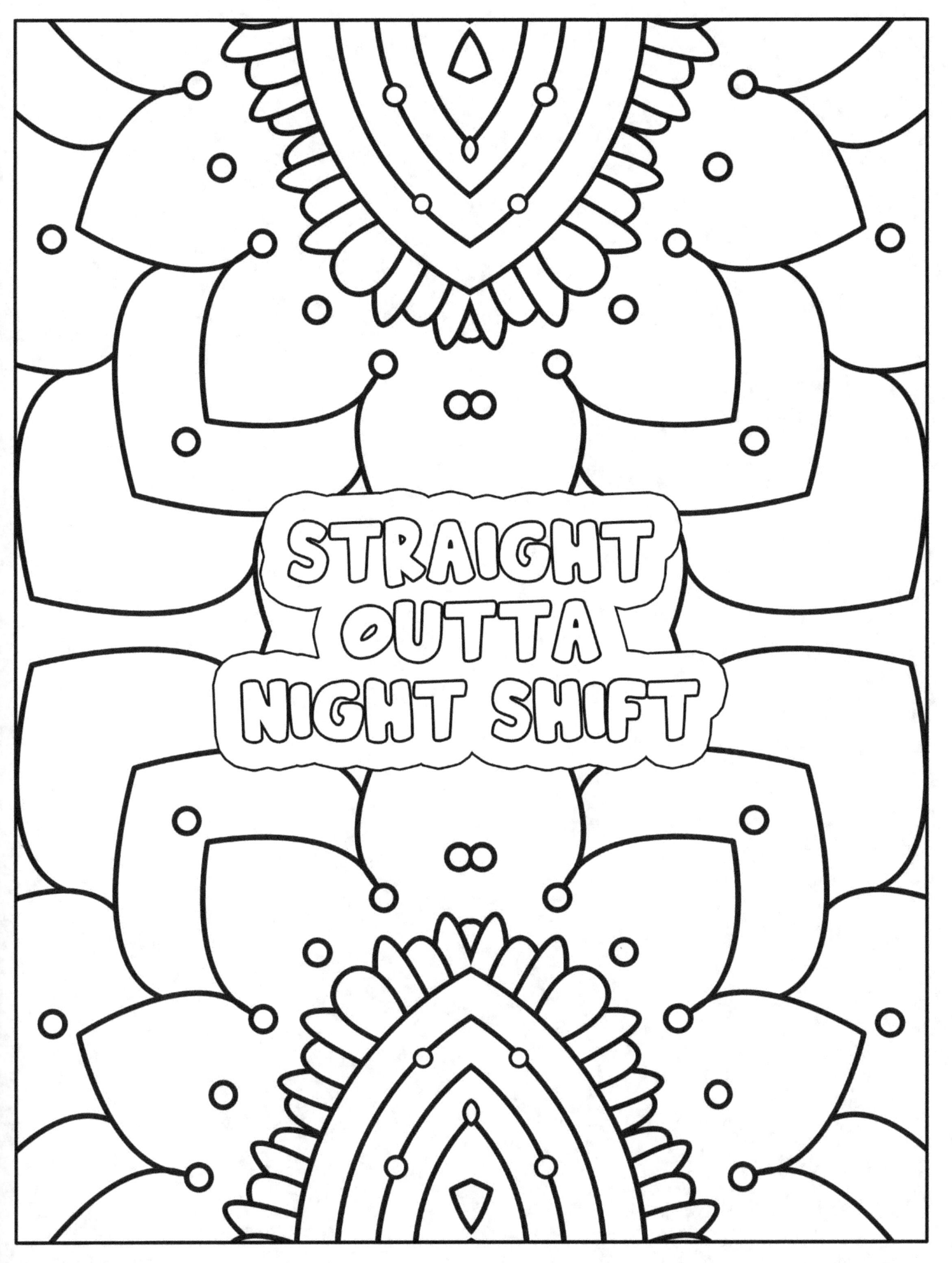

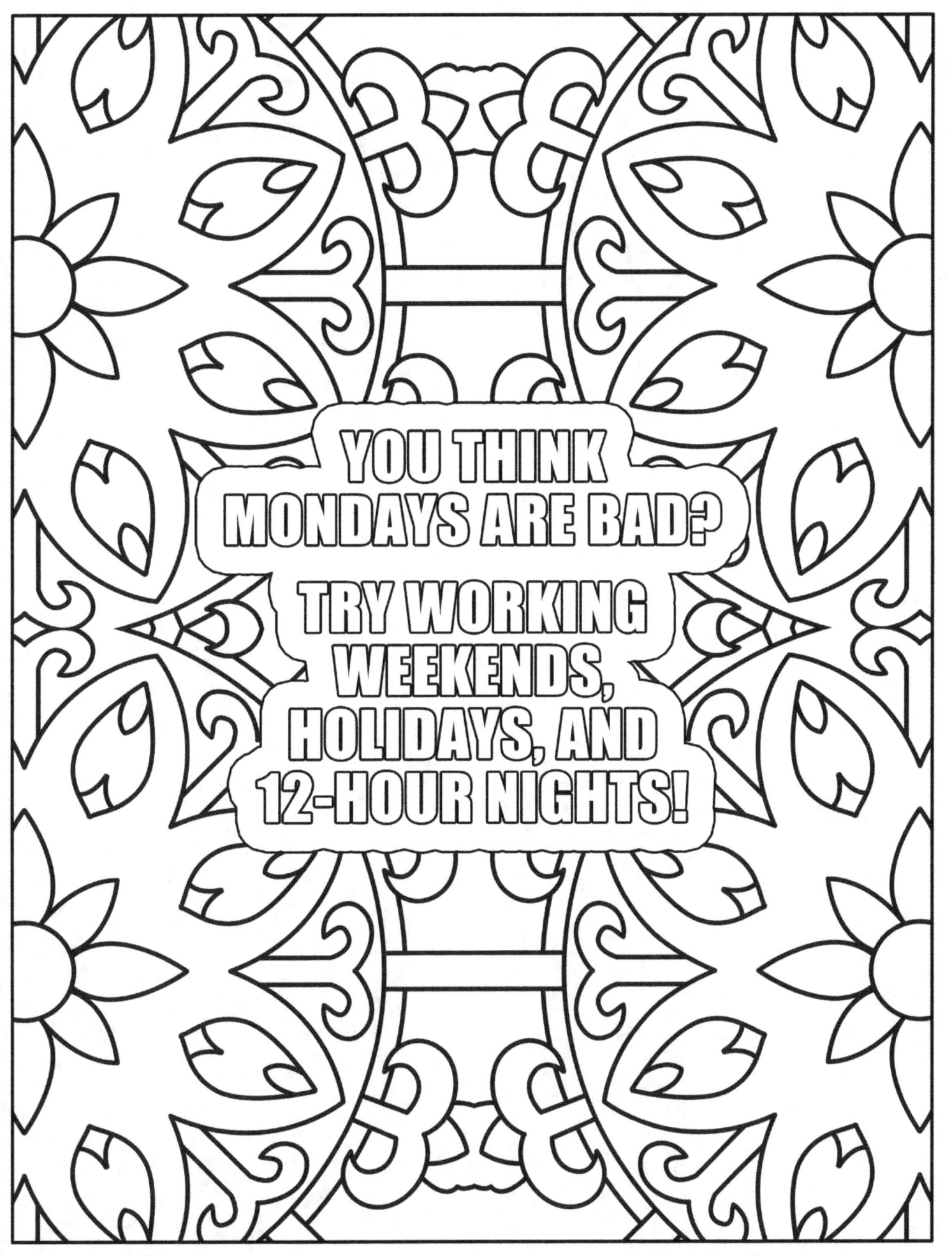

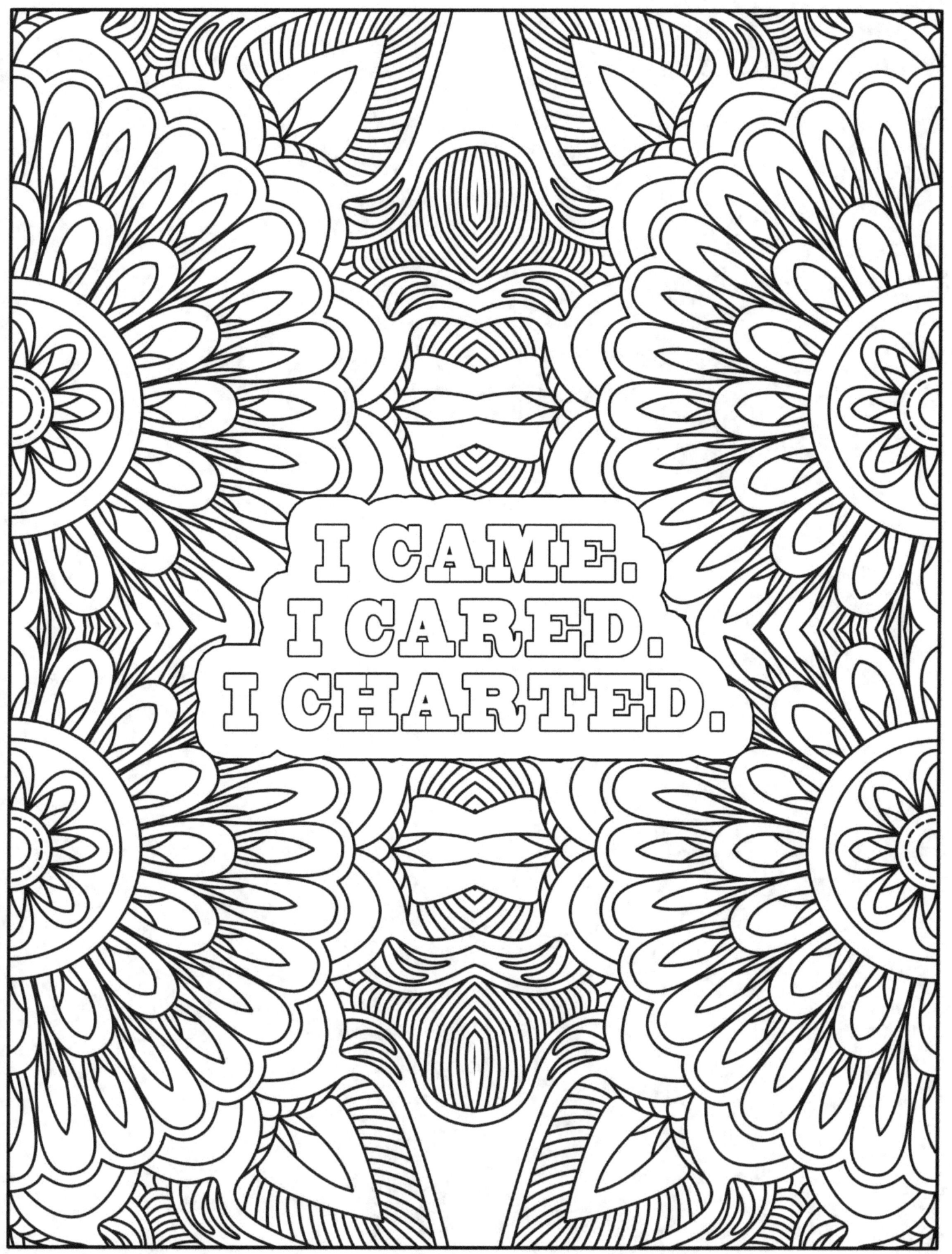

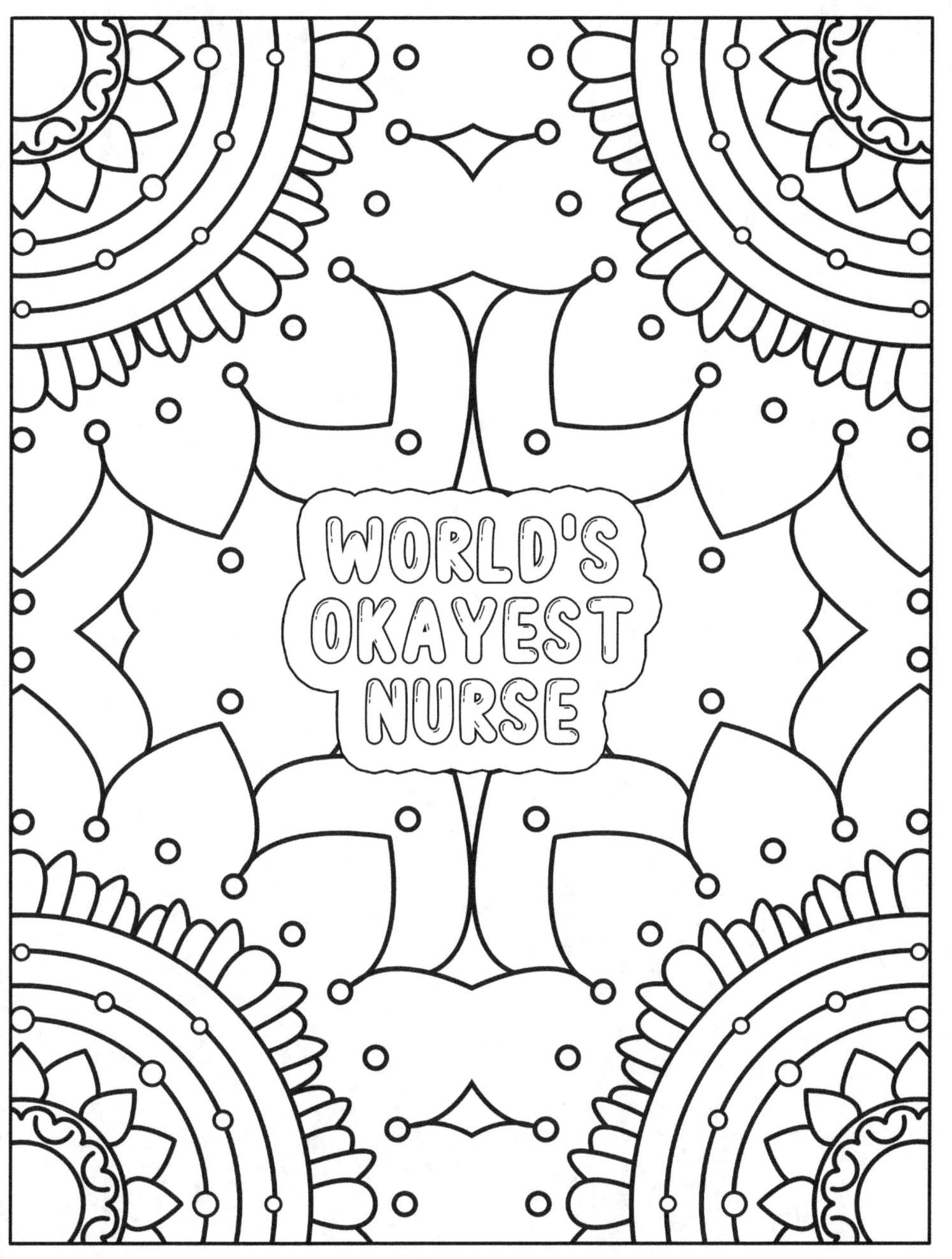

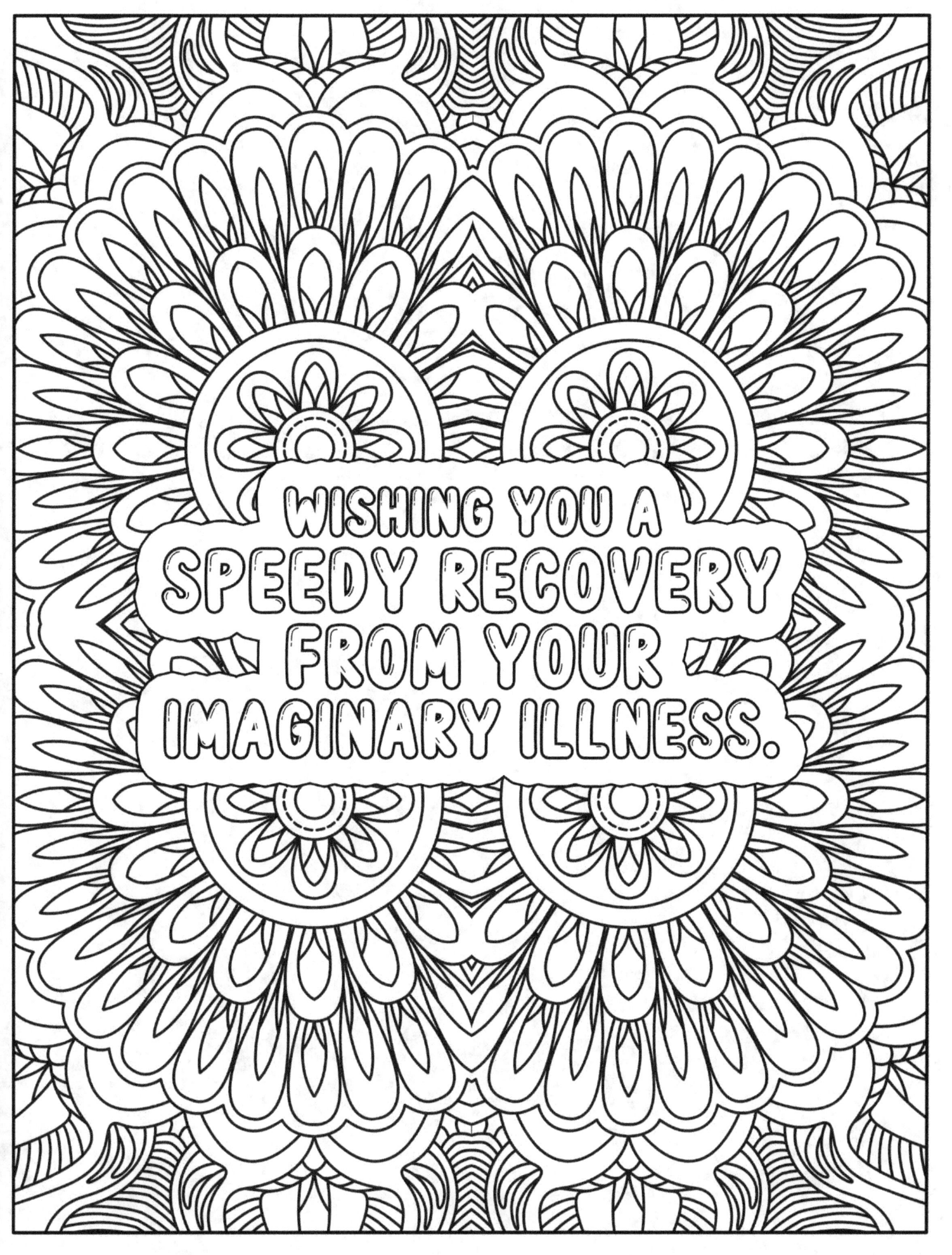

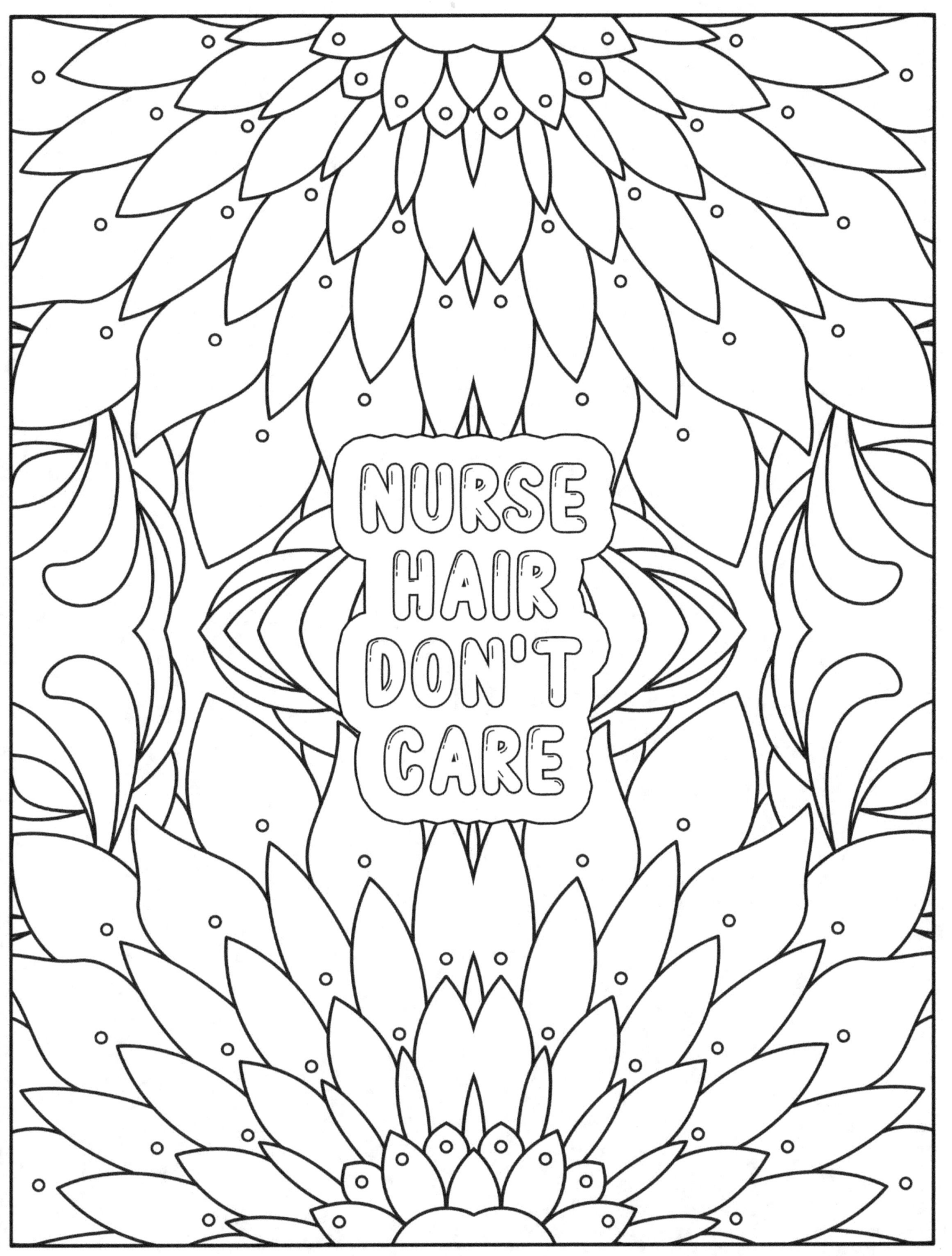

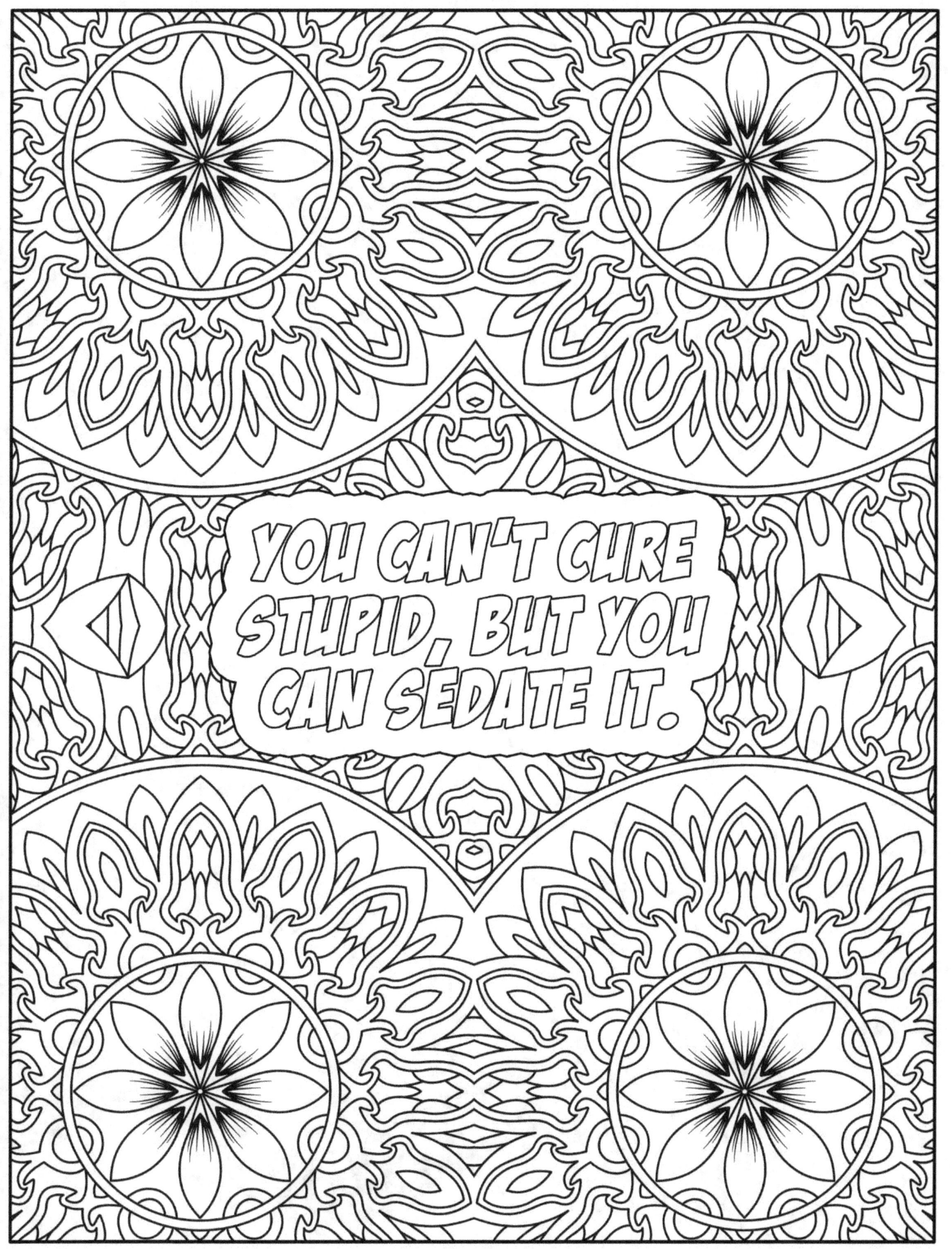

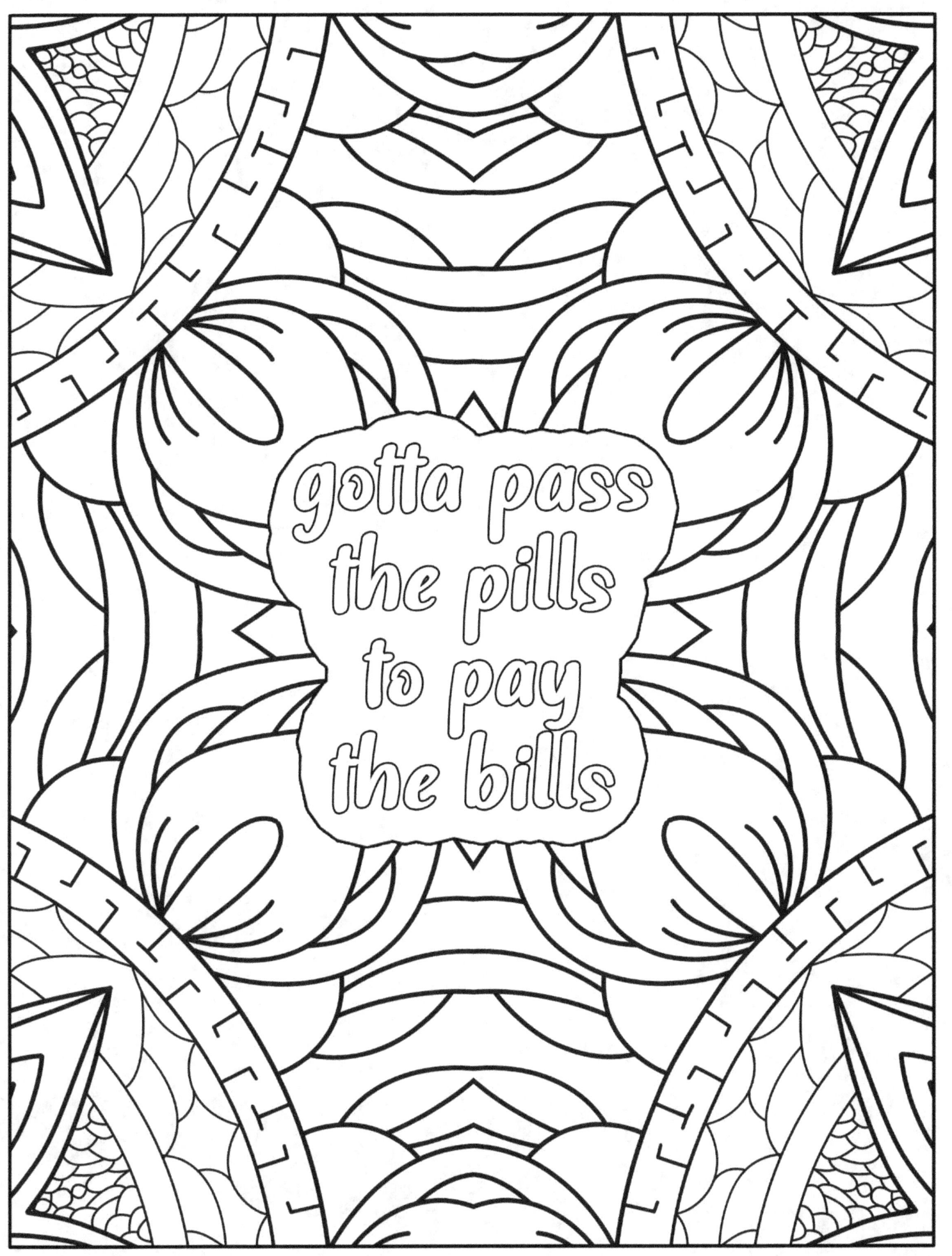

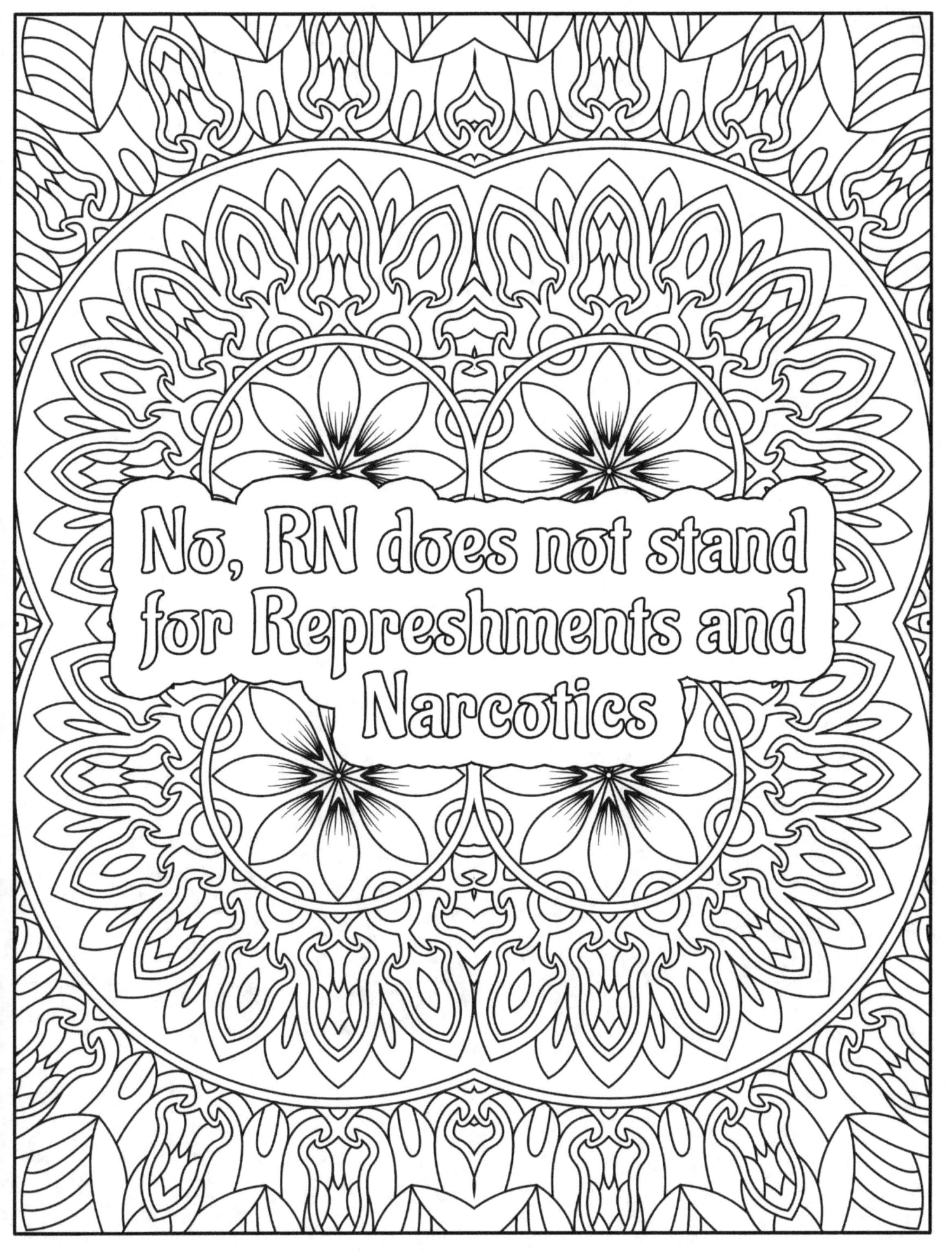

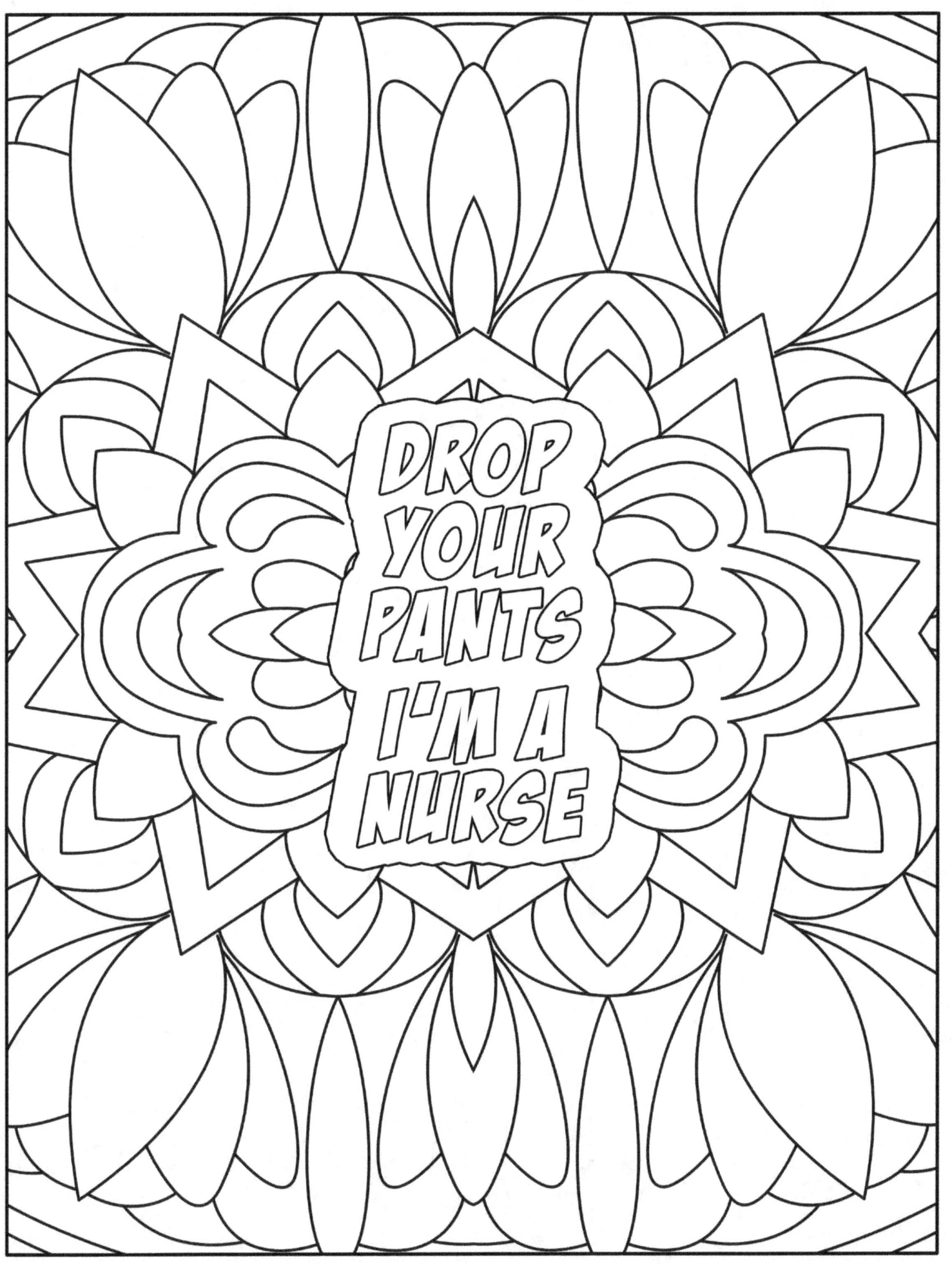

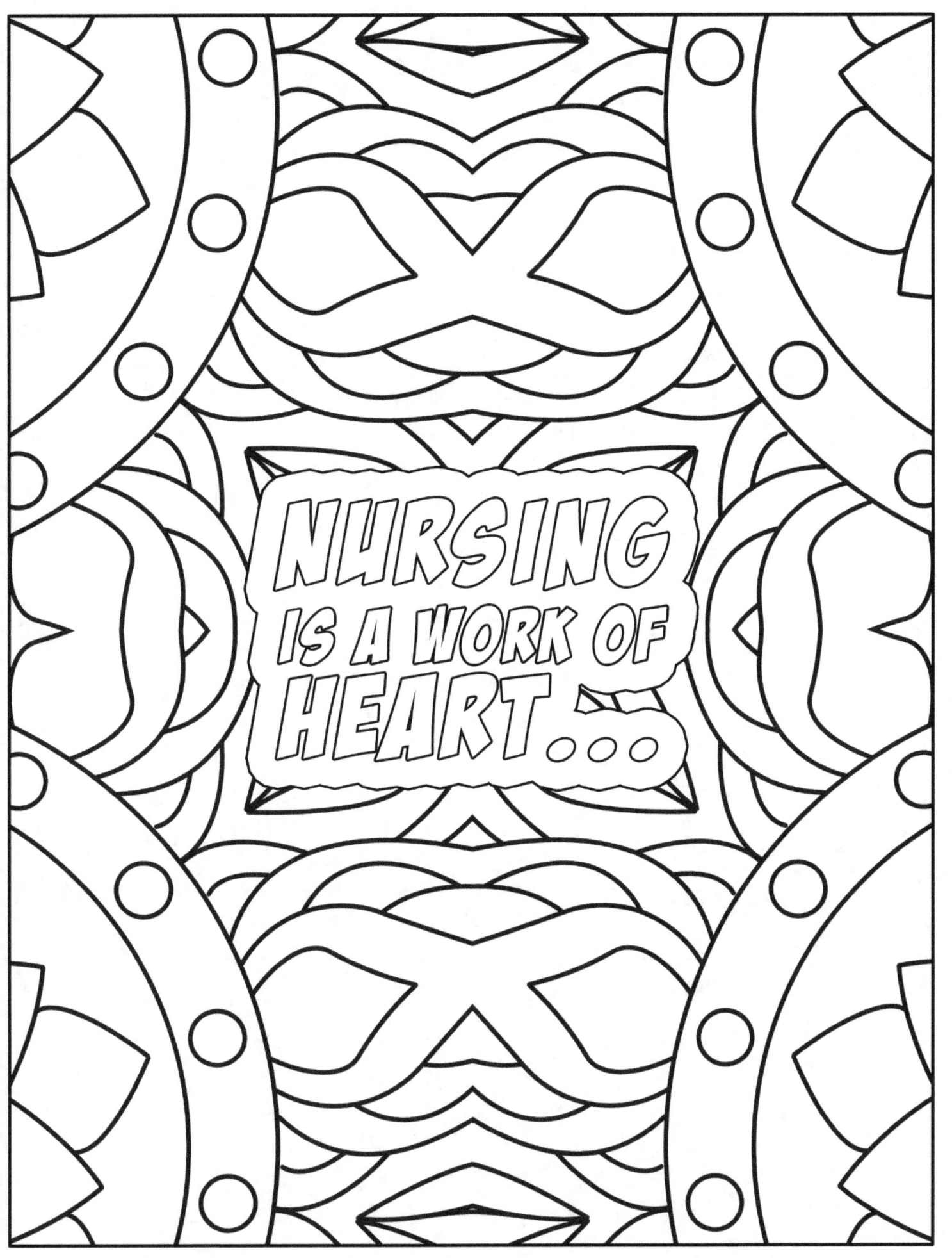

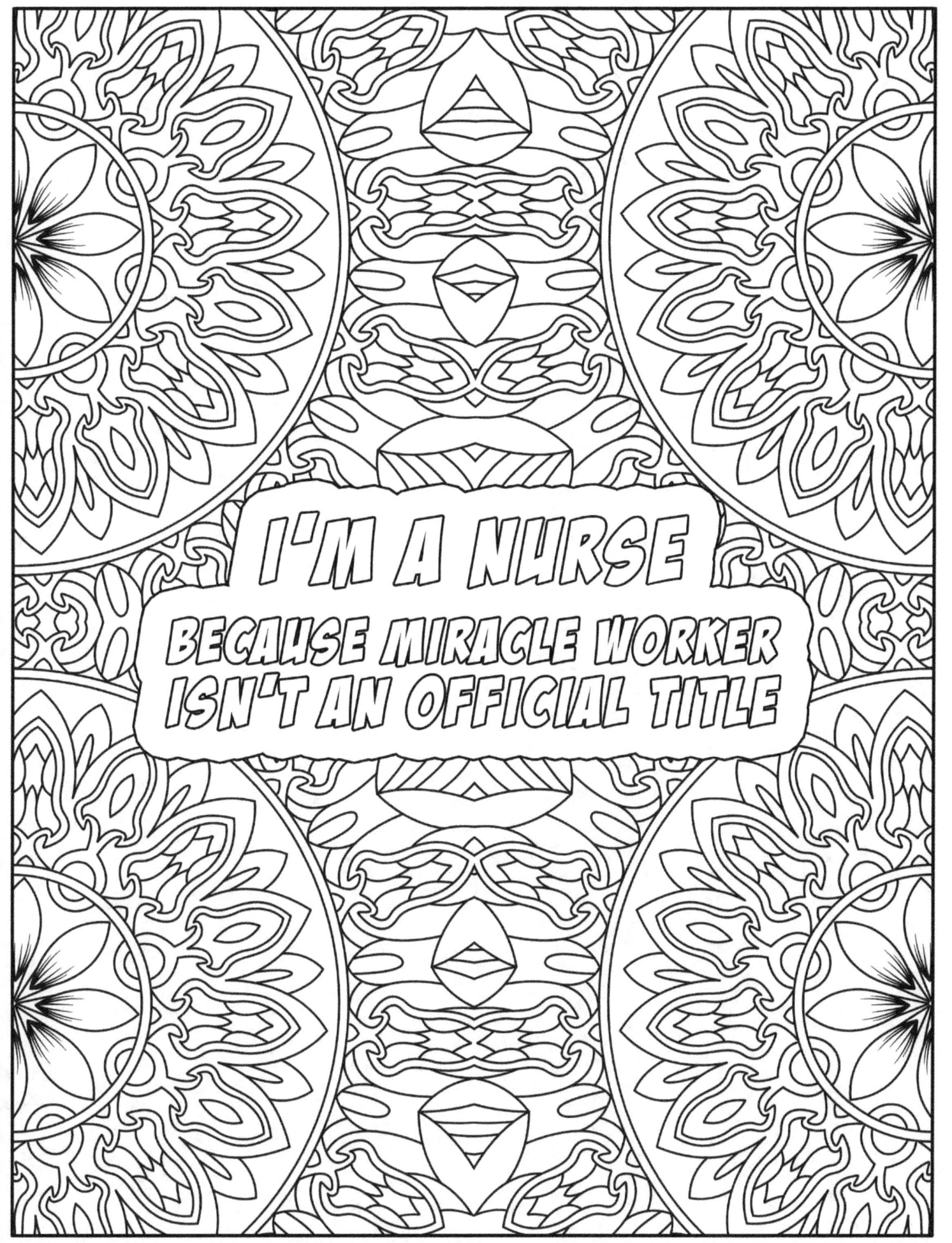

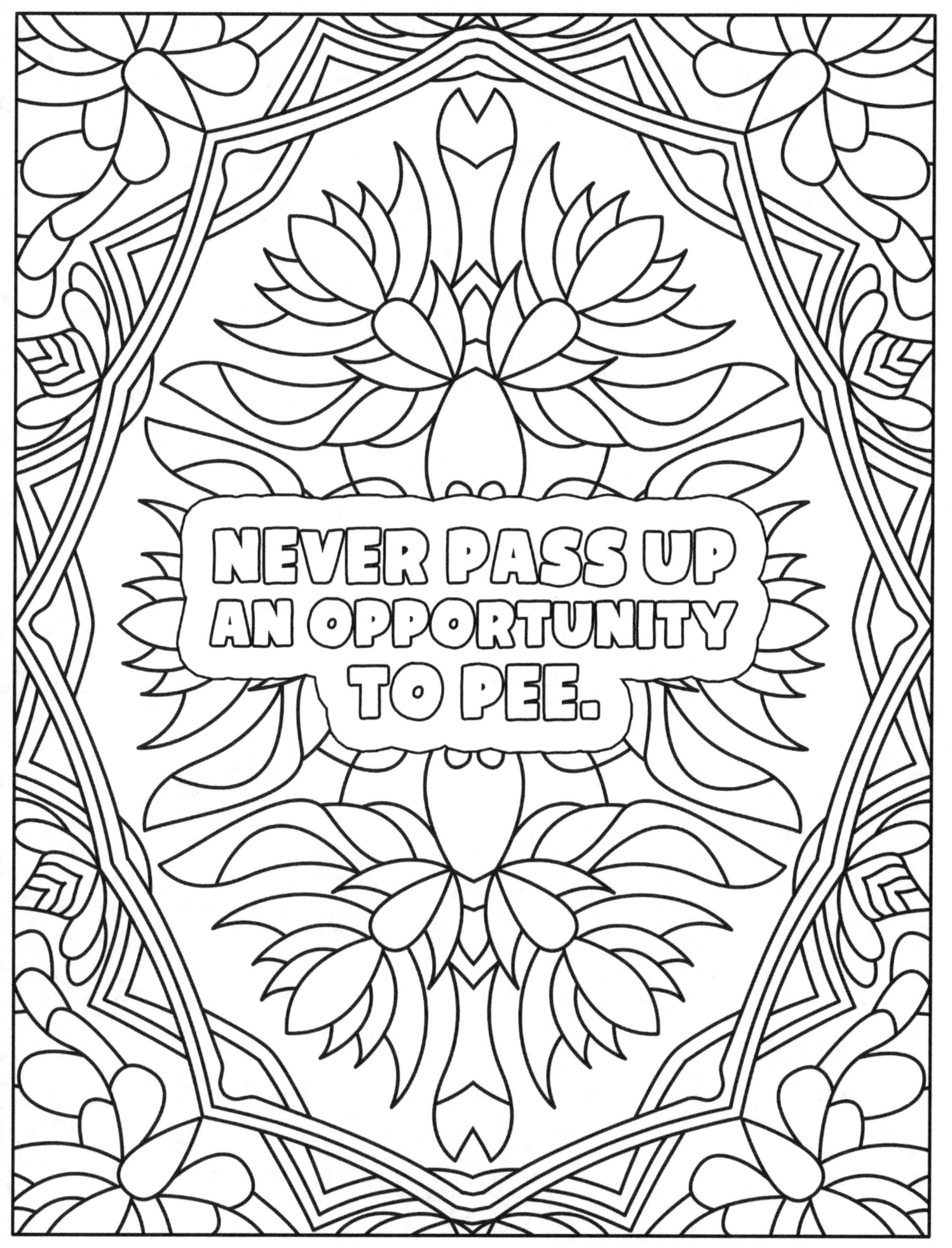

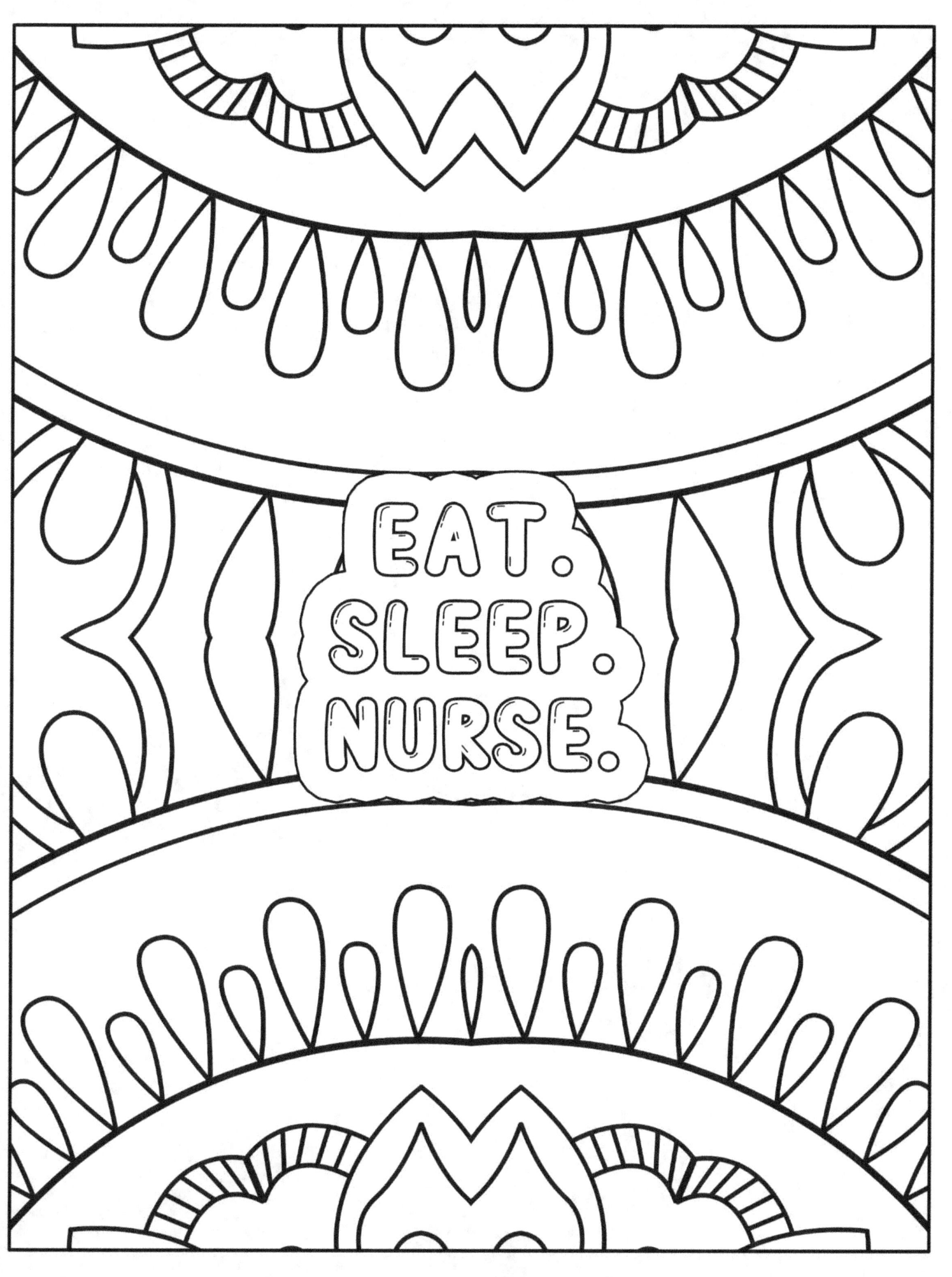

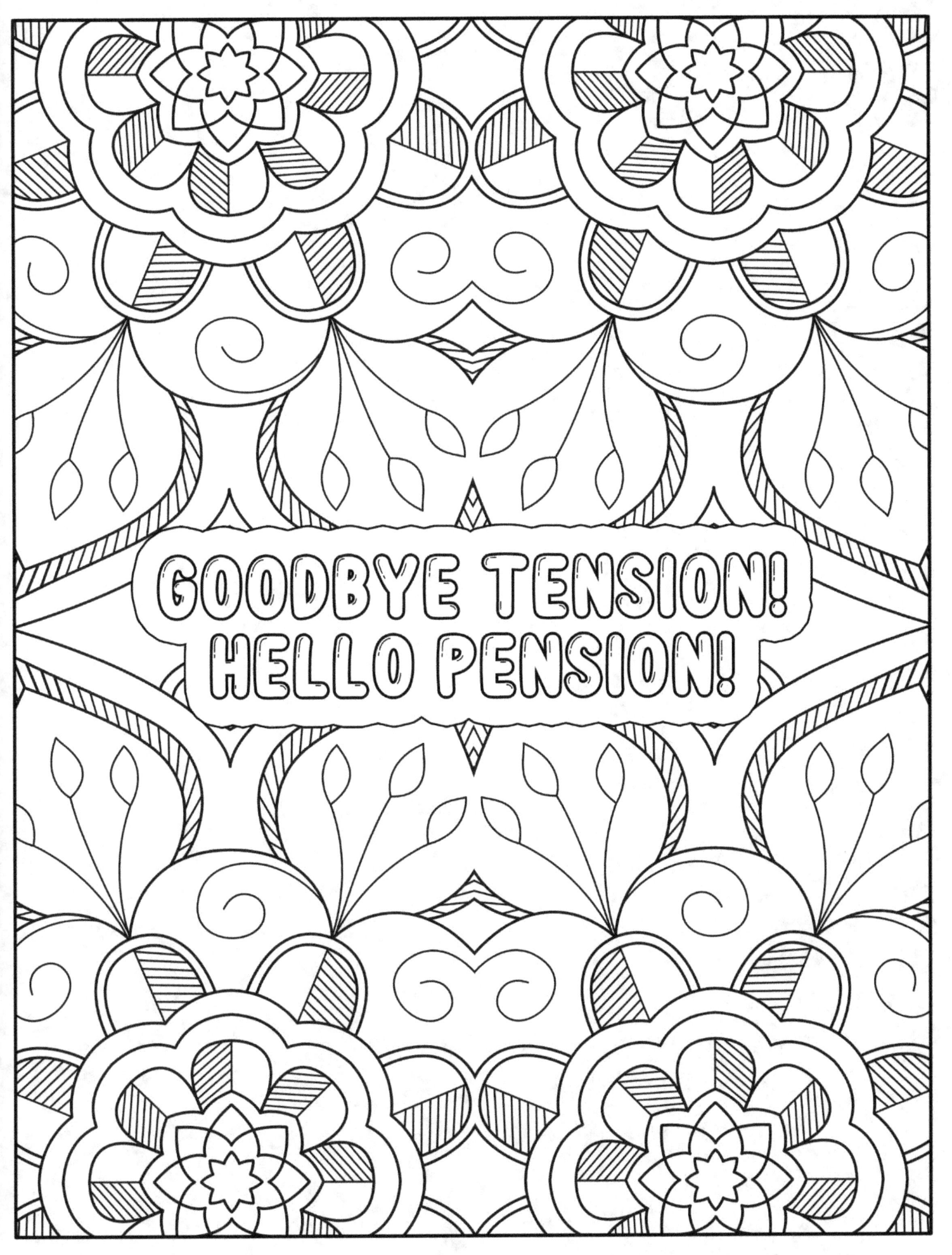

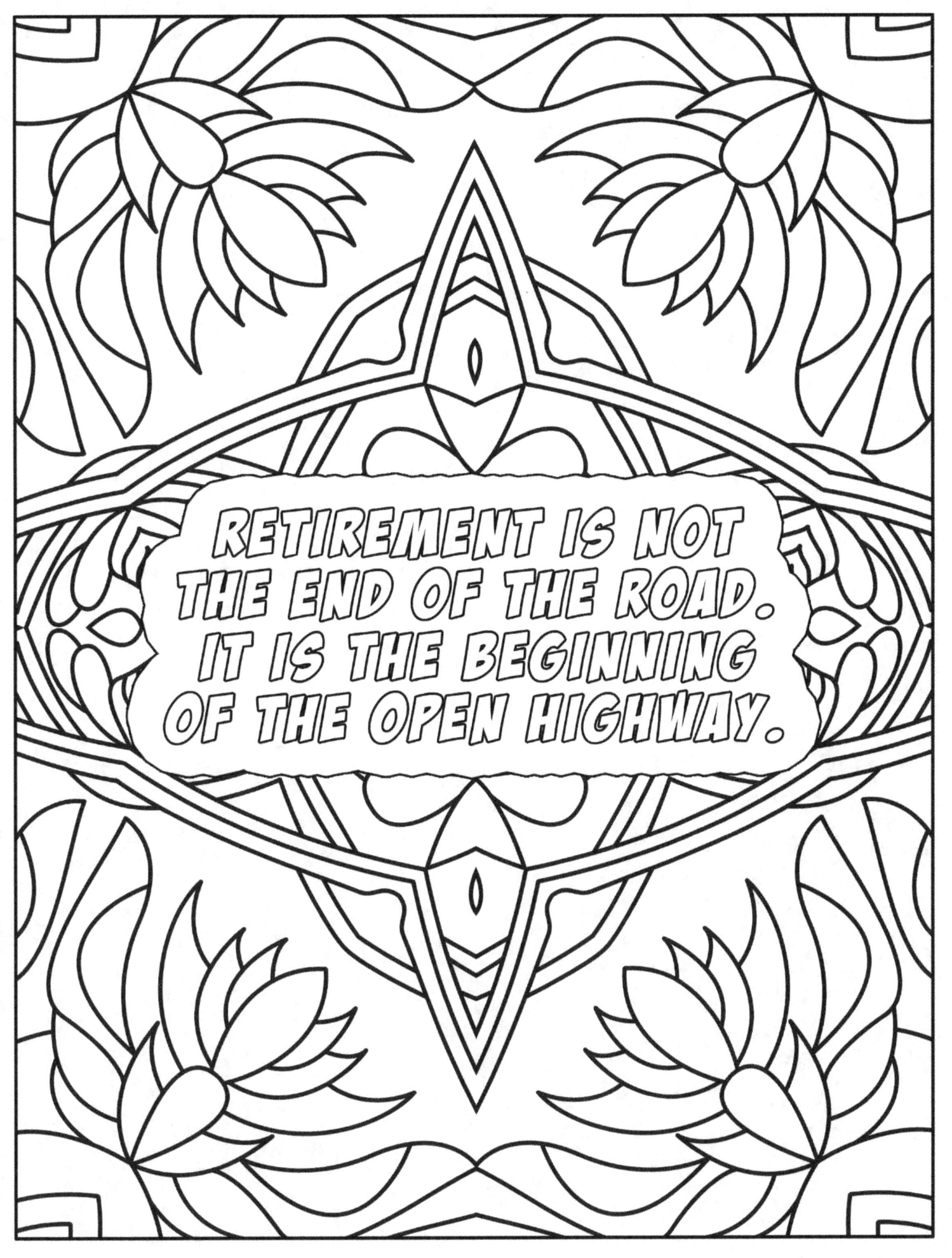

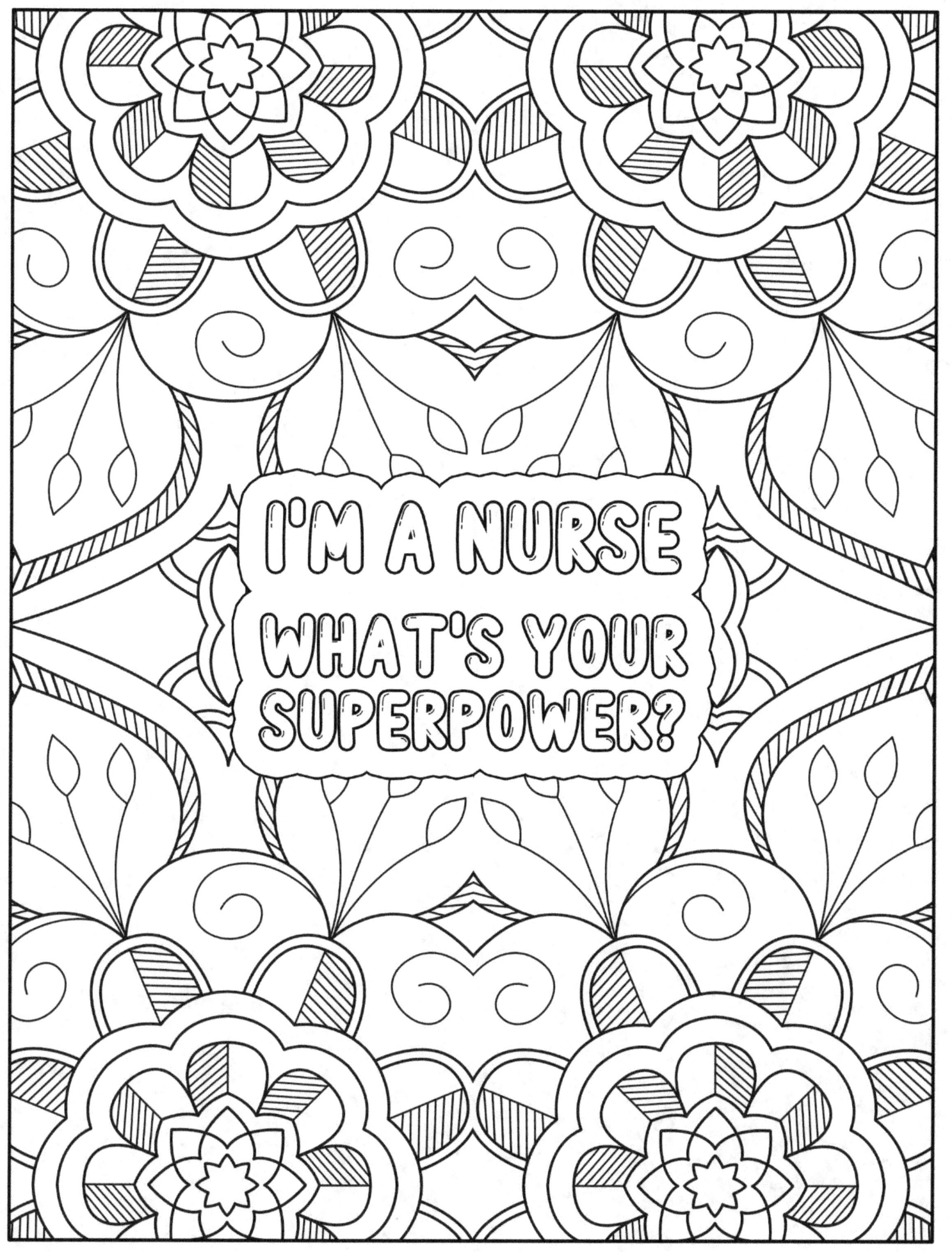

www.ingramcontent.com/pod-product-compliance
Lightning Source LLC
Chambersburg PA
CBHW080512220526
45465CB00006B/2453